"IF YOU COULD LOSE UP TO 10 POUNDS IN JUST 4 DAYS WITH FASTING* WOULD YOU TRY IT?"

Sure you would. Fasting is now a more popular way of losing weight than any other diet plan available. Why?

BECAUSE FASTING WORKS!

And now, here is the book that simplifies fasting and losing weight more than any other book ever printed.

The Layman's Guide To
Fasting
and
Losing Weight

by Phillip Partee
Edited by Dr. H. Levy Jr.
Introduction by Dick Gregory

The Layman's Guide To Fasting And Losing Weight

A Sprout Publication/1979

Published simultaneously in the United States and
Canada by Sprout Publications.

ISBN 0-932 972-00-4
Library of Congress Catalog Card Number 78-64863

Printed in The United States of America

CONSULT YOUR PHYSICIAN

It is advisable for everyone attempting to fast for weight reduction or for other reasons to first consult his physician, especially anyone suffering from serious illness. It is best that you find a doctor who is familiar with fasting and its benefits and to remain in touch with him throughout the fast.

The information in this book is not intended as diagnosing or prescribing but should be used and talked over with your doctor.

It is your constitutional right to use any of this information in a self-prescribing way but the author and the publisher assume no responsibility. No one should attempt to fast for any length of time unless he clearly understands what he is doing and also why he is doing it.

Contents

INTRODUCTION
by Dick Gregory

"Give us peace O Lord in our time."

Fasting is so beautiful, in a way it is like putting yourself on spiritual trial. Whether fasting for religious, political, or scientific (rational) reasons you face yourself with the questions, Can I do it? Am I strong enough?

The other day some cat picked me up at my hotel to drive me to the University which I was speaking at that evening; while we were driving down the road he began talking to me about fasting and how he knows it would be good for him to fast but now he's having enough trouble just cutting down from fourteen to ten meals per day, not including snacks! While he was rapping to me about his lack of self control over his own mind, he was eating a smoked porpoise stick dipped in mayonnaise and butter.

People today have been terribly misled about fasting when the truth is that a controlled fast is safe and for the most of it painless. You will soon see that most all human suffering comes from the dinner table more than from any other source. Obesity and disease are self-inflicted. America is the only country in the world where more people die each year from over-eating than undereating.

Today the food that most Americans put into their bodies is fast and fake but it ain't food let alone nature. You could look at the eating of these unnatural foods as good because the worst comes later. The real harm that comes from eating these foods is that every time you eat something unnatural, a little bit of poisonous residue is left inside your body and over the years builds up and in a way becomes you. Eating is like putting fuel in your car. As the fuel gets used up and throws its waste out the rear pipe, it also leaves a little carbon inside the engine, food alike leaves its residue inside your body. Not all food comes out!

It has often been said that what you eat you are, and it would be no surprise to me today to see bottles of chemicals with arms and legs walking down the street and big, ugly whoppers and greasy quarter pounders hanging around on the street corners. After years of being raised on a lot of this kind of food myself, and looking back and seeing how it effected my consciousness and body, I finally realized why folks pray at the dinner table over their food. It needs blessing! And I realized too that alot of the junk I had put into my body never came out. The only reason I made it through my childhood was because my momma cooked that junk food with so much love it saved us all.

After I began getting into fasting, my whole thing changed. All those nasty poisons were finally leaving my body. In fact, that is the whole health thing behind fasting, cleansing the body of all impurities, flushing out the bad food most people eat each day and giving the body a fresh start. Scientific fasting rids the body of deeply buried toxic residues that have been building up in there since we were kids, and at last once again allows your body to function as Mother Nature intended and not be chemically controlled as man today seems destined.

Another good reason for fasting is the power and high fasting gives. When you finally get that last turnip out of the pit of your belly, and your whole thing changes as you become pure inside, you will then realize just how serious of a problem eating can be and how much benefit and love not eating can generate.

My first fast was considered a hunger strike. It was mainly my personal effort in the struggle for human dignity to end the Vietnam War. Fasting I considered to have the power to be the ultimate weapon there was in the non-violent arsenal. My protest went 40 days without food, juice or prepared vitamins or other food supplements.

This hunger strike, which also turned out to be my first controlled, scientific fast, not only protested the war but soon it made me realize something else, and that was my health got better. I lost my unwanted weight. I quit drinking a fifth of scotch a day, and my two pack a day cigarette habit disappeared. Fasting started putting me in touch with Mother Nature and Her children, and who I really was. As I first began to fast, I hungered in a new way to know more about nutrition and proper food. I bought and read every book there was on the subject of fasting, along with having one of the world's top authorities there was on the subject as my personal advisor, until I developed the simplest formula to a scientifically controlled fast.

There are many books available on fasting but there are none that offer a method of fasting quite like my own and that are clear and brief at the same time. **The Layman's Guide to Fasting and Losing Weight** offers such a way. **The Layman's Guide to Fasting and Losing Weight** is easy to read, concise and brilliant, skipping the stories and testimonials, leaving only what is needed to be read. Just the short time it takes to read and study it may very well be the most profitable few hours of your life. Phillip Partee has written this book primarily to present the technical knowledge of scientific fasting to the millions of people who want to learn about fasting, losing weight and their bodies but cannot understand the complex technical data found in most books.

Phillip has properly titled his book **The Layman's Guide to Fasting and Losing Weight** as he has already done all the dictionary work of looking up terms for you.

In this handy guide you will find that each page is filled with direct, clear and concise wisdom and truth and owes much of its intelligence and direction to Dr. Alvenia Fulton who also uses and teaches the same fasting method at her clinic in Chicago. Check it out now, fast your way to not only a cleaner and lighter operating body but a higher level of consciousness as well. Find out as I have that cleaning out your body through fasting will for the better change your whole thing, the way God intended it to be.

Peace and Love — God Bless

Dick Gregory

Author's Introduction

To overcome the constant desire to eat nowadays is not easy. We are constantly thinking food.

Junk food clutters the shelves of every grocery store. Every corner has a full color billboard to blast us in the street and every T.V. screen constantly blares food propaganda at us in our homes. Promoters of the junk food industry hook the senses of the weak in the same way pushers hook drug addicts, and the danger is equal for either user.

Many people ignorant of the danger involved in the habitual consumption of these so called "foods" suffer unnecessary pain and death each year from not only obesity, but every other disease known to man.

When one finds oneself overweight or sick it is a good time to consider fasting.

In a recent survey, fasting was found to be the most popular method used for losing weight. Why? Because fasting works!

Fasting is not just another one of those "Fad" diet plans that take your money and your time. Fasting is not even a diet. There is no food consumed. There are no tablets, pills, or liquids of any kind. And it's absolutely free!

Why punish yourself with a diet plan that requires months or even years to lose just a few pounds, costs money, and in most cases, lets the lost weight come back in a short time?

With fasting you simply set your mind to lose your unwanted weight and get it over with once and for all. And when it's all over, you will stay slim because discipline is also achieved through fasting. You actually "conquer" the mental habit of eating that made you fat and miserable in the first place.

Today so many people have used fasting successfully that the myths and so called dangers have been destroyed.

Determination is the key to losing weight! If you are determined and use fasting, you too can be successful.

This book has been written with the hope of influencing people who suffer unnecessarily day in and day out from disease and weight problems, so that they may discover, as we fasters have, that the power of fasting is a gift which they can hold in their own hands without having to go to costly practitioners and institutions.

The Layman's Guide
To
Fasting
and
Losing Weight

CHAPTER 1

WHY FAST?

- To employ the cheapest, easiest and quickest way to lose one to two pounds a day
- To save time and money
- To counteract the yearly increase in food cost
- To reduce medical and dental bills by not being sick
- To give the whole system a chance to houseclean
- To reinstate the internal equilibrium of the body
- To lower high blood pressure
- To lower cholesterol and clear the arteries
- To help cure arthritis
- To help prevent cancer
- To aid in self-healing
- To prepare for surgery and for better and easier recovery afterwards
- To empty and clean the colon
- To escape from food addictions
- To break the tobacco, alcohol, or drug habit

- To calm nerves
- To become physically and mentally more alert
- To feel and look younger
- To arrest the aging process
- To make wrinkles disappear
- To eliminate and prevent acne
- To maintain health
- To free yourself from desires and attachments
- To raise your level of consciousness
- To improve your meditation
- To digest food better and regulate bowels
- To learn to eat in a healthful way
- To provide more food for the hungry
- To build supreme confidence
- To publicize political and social issues

The customary diet of the majority of American people is very near the lethal level and steadily getting worse. Counter foods (the french fry world), all snack foods and icebox foods (the shelf longevity world), and the foods for home cooking (the adulterated world) are either nutritionless, or toxic, or both. Those who eat these foods take into their system each year more than four pounds of chemical preservatives, colorings, flavorings, stabilizers, and other food additives, without considering contact with pesticides, insecticides, various drugs and alcohol, nicotine, lead and arsenic.

"Over 3,000 chemicals are deliberately added to the food we eat." (Beatrice Trum Hunter)

In the past fifty years, obesity and disease have increased very quickly to high levels here in America, higher than any other nation.

All this horror not seeming to be enough, the American eater furthers the problem through accumulating more toxic waste and mucus in the body by overcooking these already corrupt foods and then improperly combining them. Harmful food combining is typical of the gourmet eater and the Smorgasbord or buffet lover. Both styles of eating are now popularly widespread and easily accessible throughout the country. The American version of the "square meal" is another example of wrong food combining. It is "ideally" made up of meat, potatoes, bread and butter, vegetables, coffee, tea, or milk, and a dessert. This is a typical meal found in restaurants, cafeterias, in hospitals, teaching institutions, prisons, and most homes. None of these foods will digest properly when eaten together, causing in a lot of cases the protruding belly.

Even if this typical customary meal were nutritious, it is usually cooked to death and the over-mixing makes it indigestible. However, the deadliness of this way of eating is hardly recognized because there is so little concern given to the need for proper nutrition and combining. The best method is not to combine at all because one food nearly always interferes with the digesting of another. The end result of a faulty diet is the clogging and poisoning of the entire body, and obesity in most cases. When waste matter is not properly eliminated it begins to adhere to the walls of the intestines and fill the pockets in the colon causing clogged blood vessels, fermentation, and decomposition of the resulting stagnated blood. This situation gives off toxins which soon reach a dangerous level and the body sets off an alarm. This alarm can be in the form of aches, pains, upset stomach, chronic constipation, dizziness, irritability, tightness in the shoulder blades, black, or dark brown foul smelling fecal matter; offensive body odors and breath, premature aging of the skin, insomnia, dull eyes, greater need for sleep (mid-afternoon naps), eating more and more to keep up strength; addiction to sweets, headaches in the morning (or those caused by missing a meal and which are relieved by eating); stuffy nose, the constant coughing up of mucus from the throat, encrustation about the eyes, and many others, these being but some of the common ones. Most people ignore this alarm until the symptoms pass, then one day the toxic by-products build up striking you down all at once with a major catastrophic ailment. In some instances this ignoring of disappeared symptoms will have a similar effect to the ignoring of the "calm before the tempest!"

Fasting has proven itself to have an effect on disease which is the reverse of modern medical techniques. While most new age drugs and medicines result in only the suppressing of symptoms, fasting tends to bring out the cause of sickness. By not eating you actually fast out of the body suffering and disease.

"Disease and illness would be rare if every blood stream were pure, and the body was not full of waste matter and toxins." (Jethro Kloss, Back to Eden)

YOU LOSE WEIGHT

Very heavy people are never disappointed when they fast on pure water. They are often failed dieters who suffered much to lose a little weight very slowly. They also frequently regained their weight in but a few weeks. By fasting, stores of fat are broken down, burnt up, and cleared out of the body (see p. 66). Weight loss is rapid, usually a pound or more a day because all stored waste as well as fat is burned for fuel.

During a diet in which food or any outside nutrients of any kind are consumed, the process of burning fat and diseased tissues does not occur effectively or rapidly and you lose weight very slowly. Fasting is not only the ultimate diet for weight loss, but also prompts the overweight person to learn about his own body and nutrition as well.

SELF-CONTROL VS. YOUR UNWANTED WEIGHT

Discipline is achieved through fasting and the overweight person learns self-control, gaining the upper hand on his food habits, thus preventing future weight additions. Obese people not only lose fat during the fast, but after the fast, weight is also easily controlled as you will tend to eat less when the system is clean because more of the nutrients are made available when processed through a clean digestive system.

Let me make clear that fasting is not a cure of any disease or ailment. The aim of fasting is to give the body a physiological rest and full range so that the vital forces which normally would be used for physical activity and for the digestion and assimilation of food are freed for self cleansing and healing. Healing is an internal biological function. Doctors often take creidt for this natural function. A doctor can set a broken bone, but it is up to the body to mend that bone. No matter what aids one tries, whether they be health programs or direct medical intervention the body still must heal itself. Fasting gives it the best opportunity to use its force.

Fasting will help the body to more efficiently heal itself. The excretory organs are constantly expelling wastes and debris that enter the body; during a fast this process continues but becomes more efficient. By fasting, inorganic chemicals and other pollutants that have built up in our bodies, that cannot be flushed away by any other means are eliminated. Fasting is one of the most efficient natural methods of rebuilding the body's own dynamic healing powers and overcoming many major ailments. Our body is well described as being a "self healing organism." Unless disease is too far advanced, most plagued organisms are capable of experiencing a "new birth."

5

FASTING AND THE COMMON COLD

When the body accumulates too much waste material, mucus, and toxins, the body becomes clogged and choked with the excess. The body tries desperately to dispose of it in every normal way possible, but quite often fails as the excess is more than the body can handle. The result of a blocked system is commonly a cold. Fasting at this time should be employed. The cold itself is a curative process ridding the body of toxins in large amounts out of the mucus surfaces, and the fast will speed up the elimination of the mucus.

Fasting one or two days per week should be added to everyone's schedule. Whether suffering from disorders or not, fasting helps the body to help itself and is the best preventative method available to maintain maximum health. Fasting is not only the oldest method known to fight physical problems and obesity, but is also the best remedy because a controlled cleansing fast, if properly done, has no side effects as most drugs and diets do. Fasting will give the system a fresh new start, improving your future health and making you feel and look younger, breaking your attachments and desires that bind you to pain and suffering, physical as well as mental. Holy men and prophets of old have used fasting for centuries to obtain spiritual illumination and a more personal relationship to God. You will discover a power you never had before.

If you are obese, you may have more problems than you think. There are many other problems that often accompany obesity.

In the next chapter, "Death Begins In The Colon," I will talk about these problems and how fasting can eliminate them.

CHAPTER 2

DEATH BEGINS IN THE COLON

Unless you were reared from birth in a land that does not exist, where man's technology and pollution has not violated the earth, air and water, where food was grown without pesticides and sprays and hundreds of preservatives, there is a grave need for the elimination of poisons and toxins that have accumulated in your system from what you still believe is a healthy, nutritious diet; and there is serious danger if you don't cleanse yourself now. In this chapter we will learn something of what a lot of people "don't talk about," that is your bowels, and waste matter, etc.

The lower alimentary canal consists of the small and the large intestine (colon). As partially digested food leaves the stomach and passes through the small intestines (see diagram on p. 8), digestion continues; the food values are extracted and distributed by the blood stream to all parts of the body. This process is what is commonly referred to as the process of assimilation. The large intestine, or colon, then receives the

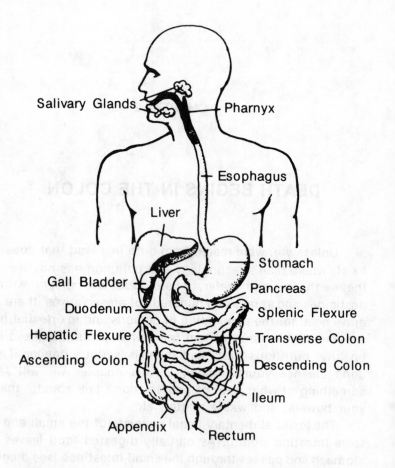

Salivary Glands — Pharnyx

Esophagus

Liver

Stomach

Gall Bladder — Pancreas

Duodenum — Splenic Flexure

Hepatic Flexure — Transverse Colon

Ascending Colon — Descending Colon

Ileum

Appendix — Rectum

The tract food takes during the digestion and assimilation process from the mouth to the rectum.

food and extracts valuable fluids which are re-absorbed and then passes waste matter our of the body.

Food that cannot be properly digested because of improper chewing, improper combination, or some other reason, will be left behind in the form of waste or fecal matter. It remains in the colon causing a fat belly and undergoing putrefaction (rotting), especially meat protein. As this residue putrefies, very toxic by-products are released, causing millions of undesirable microbes to breed in the intestines, and if not neutralized or counteracted by other "good" bacteria in the colon, (see p. 90) they can cause great damage throughout the body. If elimination does not soon take place, auto-intoxication (self-poisoning) occurs and the entire body is poisoned because the walls of the colon are porous and this poison is reabsorbed into the system. Poisonous toxins retained in the system cause the "vital energy" of your body to fall below normal. It is at this time that all of your physical and mental problems begin.

Every time you eat heavily cooked or devitalized foods, they pass through the colon leaving a coating of filthy slime on the walls much like the slime or sewer sludge cleaned out of city sewers in order to prevent them from clogging and backing up. Over the years this matter that is left on the colon walls builds up and can become so thick that the size of the opening through which waste matter passes is eventually reduced to a constricted tube as small as the diameter of a pencil. Inflamed and distorted, the colon collects wastes and fails to eliminate them, causing constipation, cancer and eventually death.

> *"Of the 2,200 operations I personally performed, I never found a single normal colon, and of the 100,000 performed under my jurisdiction, not over 6% were normal." (H. Kellog, M.D., Battle Creek, Mich.)*

Frederick A. Coller, M.D., former chairman of the Department of Surgery at the University of Michigan states that cancer of the colon now causes more deaths each year in the U.S. than any other malignant disease and that it has the highest incidence in our population of any cancer, with lung cancer second and breast cancer third. Frederick Metchnikoff, a great researcher, once said, "Death sits in the bowels."

It is impossible to find a perfect colon, one that has developed normally when diet has consisted of heavy meats and processed food. In American, autopsies indicate that only one tenth of the patients examined had a near normal colon. Most people don't even know what a colon is, what it looks like, where it is located in their bodies, and most important what its function is. (See Diagram page 11.)

"The colon is a sewage system but through neglect it becomes a cesspool. When it is clean and normal, we are well and happy, let it stagnate and it will distill the poisons of decay, fermentation, and putrefaction into the blood, poisoning the brain and nervous system, so that we become mentally depressed and irritable. It will poison the heart so that we become weak and listless. It poisons the lungs so that the breath is foul. It will poison the digestive organs so that we are distressed and bloated, and it poisons the blood so that the skin is sallow and unhealthy. In short, every organ of the body is poisoned and we age prematurely, we look and feel old. The joints are still and painful, dull eyes and sluggish brain overtake us, and the pleasure of living is gone." (V.E. Irons, Inc.)

At one time the subject of alimentary toxemia was discussed in London before the Royal Society of Medicine by many of the leading physicians of Great Britain. Among the speakers were eminent surgeons, physicians and specialists

NORMAL AND SICK COLONS

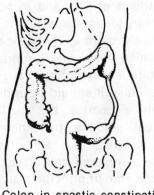

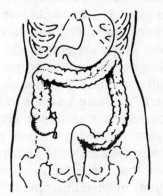

A. Normal large bowel or colon, in proper position relating to other organs

B. Colon in spastic constipation

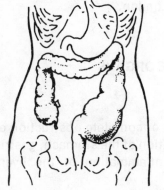

C. Colon in atonic constipation

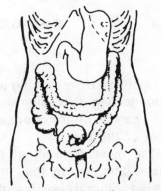

D. Psosis, or sagging of transverse colon, accompanied by displaced stomach

in the various branches of medicine. During the talks a lot of various poisons of alimentary intestinal toxemia were noted by the several speakers. One of the most commonly known, for example, is ammonia which comes from decomposed nitrogen-containing substances such as proteins and amino acids. Thirty-six poisons in all were mentioned, several are highly active, producing most profound effects and in very small quantities. In cases of alimentary toxemia some, one or several of these poisons is constantly bathing the delicate body cells, and setting up charges which finally result in grave disease. Following is a brief presentation of symptoms caused by the diseases due to alimentary toxemia. It should be understood that these findings are not mere theories, but are the results of demonstration in actual practice by eminent physicians. Of course, it is not claimed that alimentary toxemia is the only cause of all the symptoms and diseases named. Although in man it may be the sole or principal cause, some of them are due to other causes as well. In the following summary are presented the various symptoms and disorders mentioned in the discussion in London.

THE DIGESTIVE ORGANS

Duodenal ulcer causing partial or complete obstruction of the duodenum; distension and dilation of the stomach, gastric ulcer; cancer of the stomach; inflammation of the liver; cancer of the liver.

The muscular wall of the intestine as well as other muscles atrophy, so that the passage of their contents is hindered. From weakening of the abdominal muscles, other conditions are: catarrh of the intestines, foul gases and foul smelling stools, appendicitis, adhesions and "kinks" of the intestines, visceroptosis, enlargement of the spleen, distended abdomen, tenderness of the abdomen, summer diarrhea of children, inflammation of pancreas, cancer of pancreas, chronic dragging abdominal pains, gastritis, inflammatory changes of gall bladder, gallstones, degeneration of the liver, cirrhosis of the liver, infection of the gums, and decay of the teeth, ulcers in the mouth and pharynx.

HEART AND BLOOD VESSESL

Wasting and weakening of the heart muscles, fatty degeneration of the heart, low blood pressure, enlargement of the heart, high blood pressure, arteriosclerosis, permanent dilation of arteries.

THE NERVOUS SYSTEM

Headaches of various kinds — frontal, occipital, temporal, dull or intense, hemicrania; acute neuralgia pains in the legs, neuritis, twitching of the eyes and of muscles of face, arms, legs, etc., irritability, disturbances of the nervous system, varying from simple headaches to absolute collapse; mental and physical depression, insomnia, troubled sleep, unpleasant dreams, unrefreshing sleep, the patient awakening tired, excessive sleepiness, patient falling asleep in the daytime, burning sensations in face, hands, etc., paralysis, chronic fatigue, horror of noises, perverted moral feelings, mania, loss of memory, difficulty of mental concentration, imbecility, insanity, delirium, coma.

THE EYES

Degenerative changes in the eye: inflammation of the lens; inflammation of the optic nerve; hardening of the lens; cataract, recurrent hemorrhage in the retina, eye dull and heavy.

THE SKIN

Formation of wrinkles: thin, inelastic, starchy skin; (pigmentations of the skin — yellow, brown, slate-black, blue); muddy complexion; offensive secretion from skin of flexures; thickening of the skin of the back, of skin-sores and boils; herpes, eczema, dermatitis, acne, cold, clammy extremities, dark circles under the eyes, seborrhea, psoriasis, jaundice. "A small amount of poison may suffice to cause skin eruption."

MUSCLES AND JOINTS

Degeneration of the muscles: "Muscles waste and become soft and in advanced cases, tear easily." Round shoulders; flat-foot; knock-knee; weakness of the abdominal muscles causes accumulation of feces in the pelvic colon, which renders evacuation of content more and more difficult. Prominence of bones, rheumatic pains simulating sciatica and lumbago, various muscular pains, muscular rheumatism, arthritis, deformities, rickets, acute and chronic arthritis, tubercle, and rheumatoid arthritis are the direct result of intestinal intoxification.

GENITO-URINARY AND REPRODUCTIVE ORGANS

Various displacements, distortions and diseases of the uterus; change in the whole forms contour of woman; fibrosis of breasts; wasting of breasts; induration of breasts; cancer of breasts; movable kidney, floating kidney; Autointoxification plays so large a part in the development of disease of the female genito-urinary apparatus that the diseases may be regarded by the gynecologist as a product of intestinal stasis.

GENERAL DISORDERS AND DISTURBANCES OF NUTRITION

Degeneration of the organs of elimination, especially the liver, kidneys (Bright's disease) and spleen, pernicious anemia, lowered resistance to infection of all kinds, premature senile decay, retardation of growth in children, accompanied by mental irritability and muscular fatigue, adenoids, enlarged tonsils, scurvy, enlarged thyroid (goitre), various tumors and thyroid, Raynaud's disease. In those who apparently suffer no harm from constipation during a long series of years there is perhaps a partial immunity established. It is believed that such an immunity is sometimes established in the very obstinate constipation which accompanies absolute fasting because of the cleansing of the tongue and reappearance of appetite which often occurs at the end of the second or third week of the fast, a phenomenon very much like that which appears in typhoid fever and other continued fevers. It must not be supposed, however, that even the establishment of so-called immunity insures the body against all injury. The labor of eliminating an enormouse amount of virulent toxins, which falls on the kidneys, damages the renal tissues and produces premature failure of these essential organs. Any process which develops toxins within the body is a menace to the life of the tissues and should be suppressed as far as possible, and as quickly as possible.

The fact that symptoms of poisoning resulting from constipation do not appear at once is no evidence that injury is not done. One physician, Dr. William Hunter in the course of the London discussion remarked that the fact that:

> *"Chronic constipation might exist in certain individuals as an almost permanent condition without apparently causing ill health is due to the power and protective action of the liver. It is not any evidence of the comparative harmlessness of constipation per se, but only an evidence that some individuals possess the cecum and colon of an ox, with the liver of a pig, capable of doing any amount of detoxification."*

In the face of such an array of evidence backed up by the authority of nearly 60 eminent English physicians — and many hundreds of other English, U.S., German and French doctors, it is no longer possible to ignore the importance of alimentary toxemia or autointoxification as a fact in the production of disease. To no other single cause is it possible to attribute one-tenth as many various and widely diverse disorders. It may be said that almost every chronic disease known is directly or indirectly due to the influence of bacterial poisons absorbed from the intestine. The colon may be justly looked upon as a veritable Pandora's box, out of which comes more human misery and suffering, mental and moral, as well as physical than from any other known source.

Many people think that as long as they maintain their external body parts, cleaning the skin, nails, teeth, grooming the hair, and washing behind their ears, there is no need for concern about maintenance of their internal organs simply because they cannot see them. This is like sweeping dirt under the carpet.

But once informed that you have such a thing as a colon and that there is a need for constant bowel regularity and the cleansing of your insides, you cannot help thinking about your own insides and what may be their condition; am I impacted? Do I need cleaning? Out of love for humanity, I urge every adult passing the age of 45, who has not eaten naturally most of his years to have a yearly sigmoidoscopy, i.e. an inspection, through a speculum, of the interior of the sigmoid colon (that S-shaped, or sigmoid, final portion of the large intestine, just prior to the rectum) along with X-rays of the colon. The best hope for higher survival rates in cancer of the colon and rectum is early diagnosis. You may think that life is good because you have beef steak every night and eat in the fanciest restaurants in town, but at the time when discovery of cancer in the bowel occurs, you will wish that you had never listened to your mind about the pleasures of eating junk and harmful foods and had been a little more accepting of what Mother Nature had to offer. It has all surfaced now, "all natural" whole foods and habits have been presented and are recommended by thousands of authorities as a cleaner, better way of life. Failure to overcome attachment to your old way of eating can put the last shovel of earth on your grave. Your tombstone may read:

"Here lies Mr. Wish-he-hadn't, born free of mind, died too early from the evils of the mind. Mr. Wish-he-hadn't was an active member of the Diner's Club and the Fried Food Association, and was noted for his

excellence of "taste" in gourmet cooking. Mr. Wish-he-hand't was also an active member in the "Eat More Meat" and "Beef for Health" bumper sticker clubs. Now relieved of his diseased body, may his soul rest in peace."

This chapter may be the most important information you have ever read in your entire life, for these words may convince you to take fasting seriously, to cleanse yourself and someday save you from the painful experience of many of the diseases that plague mankind and which may also prevent you from experiencing an early death.

CHAPTER 3

FASTING IS NOT STARVING

Almost everyone confuses fasting with starving. While on a 40-day fast, I was approached by many of my friends and relatives who said, "You better eat or you're gonna starve." What are you trying to do, starve yourself?" This reaction occurs because people have never considered fasting in their lives and fear for your safety and health. They are unaware that fasting is a matter of choice, the choice to voluntarily abstain from food.

The faster can overcome all unintentional negativity put out by other people by determination and completely understanding the philosophy of the fasting cure. When fully understood, no amount of persuasion or ignorant concern will be strong enough to divert the faster.

The faster has the choice and the freedom to return to eating. The starver does not. Starvation occurs when a person is at the end of his rope, because food is not available, or he is unaware that the food he is getting is not nourishing his body.

The scientific faster after a few days, feels no real hunger.

His body is sustained by a supply of many days of excess tissue and resources such as mineral salts, proteins, etc., which are not available to the person who has reached the point of starvation. When the excess tissues and resources of the body are all used up, the organism is forced to feed on the vital tissues of the body organs, having gone beyond all resources is the conditions of all the millions of people who die each year in India, Africa, and all the other countries where no food is available for long periods of time.

Sun, air and water are sufficient to sustain the free choice faster whose body still has its natural resources of stored matter. In fact, one of the major purposes of fasting is the process of autolysis. This is when the body uses up these stored materials and cleanses the entire system. The body actually burns up (oxidizes) fat along with weak and diseased cells by recycling them through the body as fuel to be used and then eliminated. When this is done, the fast must be ended.

Fasting bestows many benefits. Starvation brings disease or death. That many people are misled by the confusion of these two terms is due partly to the fact that many members of the medical profession apparently do not know the great basic truth — FASTING IS NOT STARVING. The reality, and danger of this mistake is apparent in the number of times that medical men will prescribe eating for their ill patients.

> *Hippocrates once said, "If a sick person is fed one feeds the disease."*

Remember that fasting is for better health and there is no danger in it. It takes a long time to starve and the body will naturally announce to you when to start eating again before starvation sets in.

CHAPTER 4

THE NATURE OF HUNGER

The next several pages will clarify the mysterious sensation of hunger and its origin. Most fasters mistakenly believe that hunger will painfully prevail during fasting and will cause great discomfort. When most people are asked "what is hunger?" their answers are usually elementary — a cry for food or a gnawing in the stomach region. Most people are uninformed about the internal nature which provokes hunger. In order to prevent psychological stress and worry over the deprivation of food during fasting, read this chapter carefully and come to understand the real nature of hunger so that fasting can take place without fear about the need for food or fright over the play of your own organs.

To begin, there are two classes of hunger: true hunger which is physiological in its basis, that is dependent on actual bodily need; and hunger sensation, which is based in both physiological and psychological factors. Hunger sensation tends to be the less severe of the two.

True hunger is the type associated both with real pain and

suffering. Only the starving know it. It has caused crimes and provoked great greed and selfishness, suicide and cannibalism. True hunger is torment and so painful that man will go to any extreme to escape it. True hunger is an experience most of us have never known — it is not simple desire or appetite. It is much more than the common headache or gnawing stomach. Even death would not be unwelcome as a solution to this feeling, which is fortunate since this pain is starvation and death is its constant companion.

Throughout the world children die every day without ever knowing what it is like not to be hungry. Surprisingly it is through hunger that a humane solution to this suffering can be achieved. Fasting, even in a limited way, could provide enough food to feed all the hungry, and the faster could take comfort both from the fact that he is never going to experience real hunger, even though he doesn't eat, and from the good his sacrifice could do in the world. The scientific faster will not come anywhere near starving and can give his energy and his food to the relief of the world. The spiritual energy generated by fasting can create the necessary power to eradicate real hunger. The faster against hunger can repeat along with the late Reverend Martin Luther King Jr.,

"I did try to feed the hungry."

When you begin to fast don't forget that you are internally being fed. Through the process of self consumption (autolysis), the body constantly utilizes its stored nutrients. Because of this process there is no real hunger. Nevertheless, during the first few days of a fast you may think that you are hungering. This sensation is probably the result of gastric irritation and the readjusting of digestive organs that have never had a rest before and are relaxing and curling up for this nap, even if only brief. All of these sensations and activities usually disappear in two to three days.

Until all of the body's stored nutrients are consumed there is no real feeling of hunger. You won't be hungry. What you feel will be "desire" or "appetite" which is the result of psychological stimuli along with the provocation of food habit because of the contractions of the stomach's muscular wall.

Nevertheless hunger sensation and appetite are important and have effects on the organism which require our attention. Hunger and appetite are often confused but they are not the same. They are both sensations but their similarity is only that they both lead to eating. There should be no confusion of these two terms if you remember that appetite is the attraction to food and the capacity of intake — how much you want to eat and how much you can contain. This is the normal approach to food for all of us who are fed with any regularity at all. True hunger is the body's cry for help and release from pain. A person starving has no taste, and does not savor his food. He simply eats.

Appetite is tricky and causes fake hunger and even some of its more real symptoms like headache and irritability. There are no tricks to true hunger. Headache is painful and lasting and even routine effort becomes increasingly difficult. Fatigue and lassitude are constant as are restlessness and irritability. These conditions are in part caused by the absorption of toxins which the body has released. Autolysis is still going on but now the self consumption has nothing to use but poisons.

Even though we say hunger is the need for food it is not so clear how it originates. The most common view is that when food is deprived the sugar level of the blood lowers and sets off the response called hunger — in this sense appetite — but certainly not starvation. However, a German researcher on fasting, Tigerstidt, among others, proclaims that although the desire to eat is very great during the first day of a fast, the unpleasant sensation disappears early and by the end of the process the faster may have to force himself to eat. Such a result was apparent after Dick Gregory's Atlanta food fast during the week of December 25 to January 1, 1975. When the 120 participants were asked how many felt hunger after 4 days of fasting only three responded. All three went on to say that they were talking about desire or appetite psychologically caused, not true hunger.

Not only fasting but cases of fever also destroy the theory that hunger originates with lowered blood sugar, or, as in fever, the destruction of body substances by increased metabolism. Fever is a condition of increased bodily need when the sensation of hunger, even appetite, is absent. It is also noteworthy that almost as soon as a hungry person eats the sensation of hunger disappears, long before any quantity of nutrients or food value could be digested and absorbed and therefore a long time before the bodily condition, if altered by a loss of nutrients, could be returned to normal. It has also been proven that hunger can be temporarily suppressed by swallowing practically anything: canvas, leather, clay, stones, none of which would have any effect on organic losses in the body. Also fasters who keep themselves full of water report that they then feel less hungry. All of this crushes even more the theory that hunger sensation is directly the result of the lack of nutriment in the body.

Hunger may come and go many times in just a few hours which strikes further at the nutrient depletion theory. The answer to where hunger originates is a combination of the psychological and physiological. Our attitudes or habits on the mental plane lead us to food as also do actual movements of the stomach and alimentary canal. However, there is evidence that the contracted stomach and peristalsis (the mechanism of propulsion of the food mash through the intestines) do not occur when no digestion is taking place. The periods of activity last from 20 to 30 minutes and produce a rhythmic contraction of the stomach from 10 to 20 in number and may account for the continual disappearance, reappearance of hunger. Researchers Leib and Cannon have shown that the contracted state of the stomach during hunger is relieved by ingesting food to expand the stomach and this can explain why hunger sensation vanishes quickly and the ache is gone almost as soon as you begin to eat. Continued swallowing of food continues to inhibit stomach contraction. The normal adult stomach is supposed to equal the size of two fists, a little more than one pint. However, modern men and women possess stomachs often several times that of normal size. So the more stretched the stomach the greater degree of contractions.

There is sufficient evidence that these contractions provoke our hunger responses. Direct evidence was obtained by Cannon and another researcher named Washburn when they inserted a balloon on the end of a tube into the stomach of a human subject. The contractions were recorded by periodically filling the balloon with air and watching a float in a water scale attached to the tube from the balloon. The movements of the float registered all contractions of the fundus of the stomach. The records were made while the subject was fasting totally.

Between the observations of gastric pressure and abdominal movement a line was marked in minutes and an electromagnetic signal traced a line which could be altered by pressing a key. All of these recordings were kept out of the view of the subject who sat with one hand ready on the key, whenever hunger was felt.

The subject's personal report of his hunger pangs closely correlated with the record of the gastric contractions. Usually however, the contraction reached nearly its maximum before the record of sensation was started. This situation may be regarded as evidence that the contraction precedes the sensation. Cannon's work was later confirmed by Dr. Carlson of Chicago.

Researchers Rogers and Martin have examined the

stomach with X-rays and found that the essential activity underlying the hunger pang is a powerful contraction of the encircling muscles of the lower third of the stomach.

Contraction of the alimentary canal during fasting is not the source of true hunger, but is rather a display by the digestive organs of the readiness for immediate attention to foods swallowed.

So, in conclusion, what we mistake for the true hunger pang is merely a most natural occurence, not actually related to the need for food. However, contractions along with the mind's conditioned appetite almost invariably fool the average person. On a fast the feeling of hunger during the first few days being as I mentioned before, no more than gastric irritation, soon leaves. Any other sign of hunger is produced psychologically and happens most often at regular eating times. The busier your mind is at this time during the first few days of the fast the better. You can distract the mind from hunger.

However, if you feel more abrupt contractions resulting in severe hunger pangs along with the constant appearance of uncontrolled appetite these are some of the signs of the completion of the fast. However, other signs discussed in Chapter 10 will also accompany.

After reading these opening chapters you may have gotten something of an idea about hunger and your body's reactions to fasting and are now ready to learn how to do it. The next seven chapters, five through eleven, deal directly with the process and if clearly understood will furnish the details of a painless scientific fast. Skipping or ignoring any part may result in discomfort which can cause you to break the fast. Although fasting may be simple (if you stop eating you are fasting), it is unwise not to know and follow a proper method by beginning with a reduced diet accompanied by the use of the proper herbs and mechanical aids for as long as you need them. You must learn when you are ready to begin actual fasting and when you are ready to stop. Beginning may take one or more weeks and ending even longer. The following seven chapters will provide you with everything you need to know. Read them carefully.

CHAPTER 5

PRE-FAST DETOXIFICATION

To fast as comfortably as possible, prepare scientifically. Do not just stop eating and start fasting. There is a necessary drying out period, similar to "cold turkey" for the drug addict and alcoholic — in this case the food addict. This is the removal of the acid in the system left by meat, coffee, tea, tobacco and alcohol. Pre-fast detoxification of the system however, allows the faster to avoid a painful withdrawal when the fast begins. Such discomfort as occurs, if any at all, is only the sign of health being restored. The cells of your body have conditioned themselves to regular dosages of stimulants. When you discontinue giving these stimulants to the nerves and cells, there is going to be a reaction. You should also know that the fast is going to help break the stimulant habit and many deeply buried remnants of your favorite poisons will be flushed out of the system. Pre-fast detoxification also helps to avoid the sudden let down which occurs when you stop eating. Pre-fast detoxification starts the elimination and cleansing which is later intensified during the fast.

Detoxifying the system for a fast usually takes from twelve to twenty-one days. Twenty-one days seems to be the time needed by most people with a history of heavy eating and other bad food habits. In special cases up to three months of detoxifying is needed by some for long fast. The process is done simply and with various laxative herbs, raw fruits, and vegetables. No use should be made of tablets, powders or liquid laxatives, unless these are herbal. Chemical laxatives will drain all of the body's vital nutrients and increase the aging process, which none of us want. Such concoctions also weaken the wall of the intestines, reducing function and causing the user to become dependent on laxatives. Some dehydrate the body, impair digestion and cause the absorption of the A, D, and E vitamins. Chemical laxatives when taken regularly will relieve constipation but in a harmful way, and do not cure, whereas proper diet does.

There are many packaged, natural herbal formulas on the market. These are available in most health food stores. Their purpose is to aid in the elimination of the feces and the various toxins and poisons constipating body, intestines, and blood. Most are to be used twice daily, morning and evening, for the first week only. There are many other herbs also available in the health food stores which can be used in mixtures. When mixing always blend three or more herbs according to need. Herbs should not be boiled as such temperatures will destroy their properties. Bring water to a boil, remove it from the heat and add the herbs. Cover the mixture and let stand until the herbs sink to the bottom. These mixtures may be taken hot or cold and honey, lemon, or lime may be added. All drinks are best at room temperature; greater heat or cold is a shock to the system which functions normally at approximately 98.6 degrees. Mix three or more of the following for your own needs. Senna Pods, Hyssop, Gentian, Self Heal, Juniper Berries, Wild Alum Root, Wood Betony, Golden Seal, Sage, Fennugreek, Nettle, Wild Oregon Grape, Comfrey, Bonset,

Blue Flag, Burdock, Chickory, Echinareus, and Cleavers. Ginseng also has been known to stimulate digestion and is an aid to mucus elimination. All of these are obtainable at most health food stores.

During the first week of detoxification replace your diet with raw acid and sub-acid fruits and vegetables. Fresh juicy fruits and raw vegetables have a purgative effect on the bowles; do not eat bananas; they are not a juicy fruit. Fruits and vegetables that are high in cellulose, (plant fiber) such as apples, apricots, oranges, prunes, sprouts, asparagus, celery, broccoli, cabbage, cauliflower, and turnips are excellent when eaten raw aiding in intestinal elimination as plant fibers are not ordinarily chemically changed or absorbed in digestion. In other words, the fibrous food passes through the intestinal tract without breaking down. These foods when eaten raw will act as a broom sweeping clean the intestines.

Avoid eating anything that is canned, cooked frozen or dried. As you go along gradually cut down on the amount of food eaten at each meal. Do this for one week. In the next few days change the diet to only the juice of fresh fruit eliminating all solid food.

WHY FRUIT JUICES?

A diet of fresh juices during the pre-fast detoxification period enables the body to rest its digestive organs, to overcome hunger and to start the elimination process.

Fresh fruit juices provide alkali which the system requires because the organs of the body provide excess acid during a fast.

All acid citrus: orange, grapefruit, lemon, lime, pineapple, pomegranate, and grape juice are recommended.

Avoid mixing acid and sub-acid juices (see page 108) and

avoid any juices that have been cooked, canned or frozen. Squeeze your juice and drink if fresh.

Two quarts of juice and two quarts of water mixed, using only distilled water, extends the juice and is highly digestible. The diluted juice will protect you from acid and toxins entering into your system too quickly which often happens when you drink only pure, undiluted juice.

The drinking of fresh non-diluted acid fruit juice often produces a feverish condition because elimination is proceeding at too rapid a rate and throwing too much toxic material into the blood stream. Drink up to a gallon (sixteen glasses) of diluted juice daily. Continue this routine until the feeling of hunger leaves. People often refer to pre-fast detoxification as a "juice fast."

Those of you who have been on a raw food diet prior to the fast may feel comfortable by moving into the fast with just three to five days of liquid fruit detoxification. And, of course, for those of you who have eaten raw foods and fasted before, just one or two days of liquid fruit detoxification is most likely necessary.

If this detoxification period is effectively carried out, you will avoid any feeling of illness; headache, stomach ache, pain, muscle soreness, or lack of energy as the total fast begins. Followed correctly, this method insures that you have gotten off to a good start on your fast and can avoid feeling day to day stress. When you move into the water fast, the body takes over the process of elimination which you began and continues your cleansing. The cleaner your system is of acid because of effective pre-fast detoxifying the more easily you will be able to fast for any length of time you need.

Anyone who feels miserable from being overweight will on or about the third day begin to notice a feeling of lightness. That bloated feeling will already be on its way out. Those with high blood pressure will also begin to feel exuberant as the arteries become free from obstructions, all of which is just the start of a whole new experience caused by being released from the harsh poisons and fat found in the typical American diet. You will quickly, and for the first time, begin to know the power and the pleasure of fasting.

CHAPTER 6

HOW LONG SHOULD I FAST?

The length of time that you should spend in a cleansing fast depends on your individual condition, how bad the body has been abused, age, (usually the older you are the more toxic you are), and previous diet, types of drugs previously used, nature of illness (if any) and how much of a desire you have to help yourself.

Throughout this book, I refer to a short fast as one of anywhere from one to twenty-one days, and the long fast being that of twenty-one days and more. In most cases good cleansing is obtained in twenty-one days.

In a lot of cases, series of short fasts are preferable to the longer fast. It is not always possible for the elderly, the working and the chronically ill to fast for long durations; but note that the "crisis period" the time when discomfort, if any, is felt during a fast is the first few days. Therefore when doing a series of short fasts, don't let an early bit of discomfort discourage you from again using fasting. The short fast is very effective and valuable. Almost invariably, fasting becomes

33

much easier after two or three days.

Thin people usually do not need to take long fasts, unless there is a special problem that needs correcting. The thin person in most cases has not abused the body by overtaxing the system as have obese people. Also, the better nourished the faster is at the time of the fast allows more fasting time. The poorly nourished individual cannot fast as long. During fasting most of the food reserves which are not used right away for energy are stored in the adipose tissue as fat. Since fat is capable of being stored in large quantities, obese people can withstand a longer duration of time. The overweight person finds it much easier to go without food. The loss of weight causes absolutely no fear making the faster's mental attitude positive, whereas psychological barriers will quite often be set up in the already thin faster when he becomes slightly thinner. Physiologically speaking, for the overweight the shorter the fast, the less weight is lost, and the longer the fast the more weight is lost.

I might mention also that the thin person cannot go out of control losing weight during fasting because the body just does not do that. You will not lose beyond what's normal. You would have to have a wasting disease in which the cells and tissues die off to go beyond the normal weight loss whether you are eating or not, or you would have to ignore the breaking signs.

The thin person who has always had trouble gaining weight will notice after fasting as the digestive and assimilation system of the body is rejuvenated, that weight will easily be gained without stuffing the body with fats and sweets. Eating of fattening food to gain weight was just defeating the purpose. High calorie foods clog the body thus preventing any nourishment from better foods being assimilated and utilized. As the system becomes clean of all obstacles through fasting, nutrients will be absorbed into the body and not flushed out of the system.

One of the best preventive measures taken against

disease and obesity is a fast of one or two days every week. Why wait until illness strikes, it is much easier to clean and rest the body every week and rid yourself of accumulating poisons than to let them build up. One or two days, however, is usually not sufficient enough time to cure a chronic disease. Chronic disease however can often be gradually overcome by a series of several short fasts as fasting does have an accumulative effect. This will enable the chronically ill person to slowly eliminate the toxic waste matter responsible for his illness without seriously interfering with normal body functioning. It is also better for older people to take fasts periodically than to take a longer fast.

There are as many different lengths of fasts as one can invent: the non-breakfast plan, one half day fast, one day fast, weekend fast, seven, fourteen, twenty-one, twenty-eight, and forty days.

Most people fast every night and don't even know that they are fasting. They go to bed every night and continue until the next morning without eating, providing they don't wake up for a midnight snack, then upon awakening they break the fast with BREAK-FAST. During this time the digestive tract gets a much deserved and needed rest; however, many systems are overworked throughout the night trying to digest that steak from dinner especially when eaten late. People ignorantly abusing and overworking their systems with too much of the wrong foods is a widespread failure of our generally good common sense.

THE SHORT FAST

For those of you who have never fasted before, try a few one to three day fasts with the proper detoxification. Detoxifying will help you to prepare and gradually ease you into a more comfortable feeling about trying the fast of longer duration. The more often you fast — the longer you will be able to fast. Space these short preparatory fasts out one or two weeks apart and replace at least one or all cooked meals with live food like raw fruit and vegetables.

Weekend fasts are excellent and are preferred by many. In most cases the faster also has the weekend free from school or work and can more easily go off to be alone, away from the temptations and aggravations caused by friends, and cooked food and its odors.

THE LONG FAST

For the longer fast, never set a time limit. Long fasting should never be considered a feat of endurance, but rather should be taken more seriously. Let developments determine the length of the longer fast. It is very unlikely that you will fast too long by mistake, natural signs, which are discussed in Chapter ten will definitely tell the faster that his fast is completed. For those of you who are suffering from chronic and acute disease, fast until the natural hunger of the body returns.

Everyone adpats to fasting in a different manner. If you have a medical problem and have been using drugs, always consult your doctor before fasting, especially if you plan to fast more than 21 days. Naturopathic doctors are good advisors in most cases.

It is not fair to the faster of long duration, 21 days or more, to continue to work or carry on with daily chores. A considerable amount of bodily vitality is consumed while the body throws off years of toxic waste materials. However, fasters of short duration, (one to twenty-one days), if your work is not too demanding, you can continue without a problem.

Vacation time is a good time for the longer fast; however, for those of you who now suffer from symptoms of acute disease (impaired health) waiting for vacation time to roll around could prove harmful. Impaired health should not have the chance to become worse and fasting should be employed as soon as possible.

In all cases of fasting where there is an indefinite period of time, and where fasting is controlled by day to day developments, your body will automatically let you know how long to fast.

PUBLIC AND RELIGIOUS FASTING

In cases of public fasting for political reasons, better known as a hunger strike, there is no limit. When people get together and fast for a reason it may take a long time to settle the issue. Once an Italian political prisoner fasted until his death for what he thought was right. Whether the problem is political or personal, it is nothing a fast cannot cure. Fasting can solve medical problems, financial problems, lover's quarrels, and even major wars. Religious fasting can be both for heightened spiritual awareness or as a means of penance for past sins. The time limits can vary and usually do not deal with the body's reactions.

Whatever the length of or reason for fasting, join the thousands of folks who fast one day a week from Friday at 6:00 p.m. to Saturday at 6:00 p.m. This one day per week was permanently organized by Dick Gregory as not only an effort for health but also to raise the energy level on that day so that the energy can be directed toward solving problems everywhere. Friday is also the day of the Christian fast, as the day of Christ's death. The energy of one person fasting is powerful and the energy of 50,000 is beyond the mind's comprehension. When we get the entire country fasting together one day a week, the power and energy level will be so high that on that day no problem will go unaffected.

PEOPLE WHO SHOULD NOT FAST

Fasting scientifically never made anyone sick, however, some conditions make it unwise for certain people to attempt to fast, without your doctor's approval: among them are heart disease, kidney diseases, liver diseases, cerebral diseases, diabetes, active pulmonary diseases, cancer, blood diseases, gout, tumors, bleeding ulcers and people taking medications. In cases of extreme emaciation a doctor's guidance is also needed.

CHILDREN AND FASTING

Children should never be forced to fast or to eat. They have a better instinct about the matter than most adults do. They know instinctively when to fast and for how long. This is why when a child refuses to eat you should not force him. There is a reason for not wanting to eat. Children as well as adults, lack desire for food when ill. Soon the appetite will return. But in the meantime you may do damage to the child by forcing him to eat. Parental mistakes in the child's nutrition are often the cause of the child's disease. During their formative growth years, children who are healthy should never be fasted.

THE WEAK AND FASTING

The weak should not hesitate to fast. Their weakness is most likely due to toxemia which can be eliminated through fasting and not lack of food. Usually the weaker you are, the more need for fasting there is. Women who have just given birth to children must not fast. It is alright for a pregnant woman to fast for very short periods, during the first few months of pregnancy under the direction of a doctor qualified and knowledgeable about fasting. It is nonsense to believe the expectant mother must eat for two.

It has been said that "Mary fasted before Jesus was born and kept things hid in her heart."

Thin people should never hesitate to fast. It is a mistake to think that only the heavy can safely fast. It is only when emaciation is extreme that any special caution should be necessary.

SENIOR CITIZENS AND FASTING

Older folks should never hesitate to fast, but only with their doctor's approval. By using fasting, older people will feel younger, become more active, and live longer.

CHAPTER 7

THE IMPORTANCE OF COLONIC HYGIENE

Most people don't like enemas. I don't either; however, when faced with the internal recirculation of poisons and waste matter, the enema becomes more acceptable. Life seems to be full of unpleasant things made necessary by the neglect of other things that should have been done in the first place.

A clear understanding of the enema's function can be seen by example. When you use a radiator flush in your car's radiator it breaks loose all of the dirt and rust within. It would be of little use after loosening all of that debris not to flush out and drain the radiator. Of the body the same thing is true. Fasting with the aid of enemas, loosens the impacted fecal matter in the colon which has been storing toxins and poisons for most of our lives.

The cleansing enema flushes clean these wastes. During fasting if the enema is neglected autotoxemia (self poisoning) often occurs, especially because natural stimulation of the eliminative reflex (waste matter pressing against the rectum) is not present, adding to the retention of the released impurities, acid and mucus. In other words, after the last meal is digested, the digestive track becomes inactive and there is hardly any bowel action. Bowel movements are infrequent or altogether absent during fasting.

By autolysis dead cells and diseased tissues are being burned and the toxic wastes so long accumulated at this level also are loosened. Both are expelled via the digestive and alimentary canal and all eliminative systems. These are normally the main pathways to eliminate toxins from the body, but with the stopping of natural bowel movements, this pathway is closed without the use of enemas. Without the daily use of the enema during fasting you often experience a good deal of discomfort — headache, weakness, cramps of stomach and muscles, great fatigue — and you can become seriously ill. There is no other way available for anyone to obtain such quick relief from headache or other aches and pains caused by metabolic disturbances than through the cleansing of the colon with enemas.

> *"Colon hygiene combats the beginning of decay, pro-pagation of disease germs, and the spreading of toxin at the very source, from a purely functional point of view, the greatest amount of discarded waste is dumped into the colon. Since there is no bulk connected with this excretion, contractile movements of the gut can hardly be expected. The resulting dormancy in the intestine does permit some re-absorption of the highly toxic material into the blood stream, often explaining severe headaches experienced during the fast."*
> *(M.O. Garten, D.C.)*

The enema will wash out this constant source of autointoxification; to resist it because of a feeling of distaste or fear is unwise. If you don't take enemas don't fast. The enema then permits the faster to escape all of these pains and fast in safety.

The cleansing enema or "internal bath" is no more than bathing yourself internally just as you wash the external body. The standard enema is a remedy anyone can perform at home. The enema bag may be bought at any drug store quite cheaply. Many are also hot water bottles with plugs and attachments for both enemas and use as a warmer. The standard enema bag has a two quart capacity which is the usual amount needed although some authorities recommend using four quarts. There is usually less discomfort and greater ease using just two quarts.

HOW TO ADMINISTER THE ENEMA

The content of the enema should be only lukewarm water slightly below the temperature of the blood, without salt, soap, soda, or any such additive. The use of the strained juice of one or two lemons or limes and a tablespoon of blackstrap molasses may be added. Lemon is a cleanser in this form just as it is when taken by mouth, and the molasses is a source of B vitamin that helps counteract nervousness and rectal stress which sometimes occur when doing the enema.

Hang the enema bag no more than 2-2½ feet above you for the proper rate and pressure of the flow. Any higher may be painful. If there is no hook available to hang the bag from, do not forget the bent coat hanger and types of suction hooks are available in most hardware stores, often helpful to the person who travels a lot.

There are several positions in which to take your enema. Some people prefer to kneel while resting the head on the ground or a forearm with rear up, others like to like to lie on their left side with the knees drawn up, like a fetus. You will discover what is best for you by trying. Yoga offers many positions which work well, such as the candlestick position or head stand.

After setting up the equipment the tip of the tube should be lubricated before being placed in the rectum. Any natural oil is acceptable, but no petroleum products as they damage mucus membranes. Olive oil, K-Y surgical jelly, or if nothing else your own saliva will work (do not use soap).

Before inserting the enema tip open the tube and allow some water to flow in order to be sure that there is no air lock in the tube. Also the presence of air causes the immediate urge to eliminate and causes discomfort.

When the water first begins to enter the colon there is occasionally some discomfort. The feeling usually goes away and the enema is readily completed. If discomfort persists or is too great, never hesitate to stop and let the water out and simply begin again. Enemas are never harmful under normal circumstances. If, in the beginning, the entire enema is not accepted into the colon, the two quarts may be taken in stages.

Once I supervised the fast of a very overweight man. He was unable to take in water even in a small amount because his colon was so obstructed. So he underwent much more detoxification using herbal laxatives which softened the stubborly hard feces and soon he was able to take in water which quickly increased to the two quarts.

The enema tube is usually furnished with a small movable clamp which allows you to open and close the tube. It may also be used to control the rate of flow into the colon by pinching it. Sometimes it is only the rate of flow which causes discomfort, but this is easily avoided.

After you have let all of the water in, you should retain it at least fifteen minutes to allow the water to have a softening effect upon the feces and to carry away as much of it as possible when the water is expelled. Use five minutes on your right side, five minutes on your back, and five on the left. In each position massage the colon, and ascending and descending sides when lying on your sides and the crosstop — in the transverse colon — while lying on your back. (See diagram on page 11.) The massage should be gentle but firm. It is a considerable aid in working the water through the colon.

Fifteen minutes is usually long enough for the water to have its dissolving effect in the colon. After the water is released, return once again to your left side massaging the descending colon once more. In most cases another urge to release more water will take place. This will insure you that the colon is completely empty of water.

After the water is eliminated you may notice an increase in urination. This usually means that some of the water has been absorbed from the colon into the kidneys. This absorption can be cut down by consuming a pint of water a few minutes before the enema is taken. This will furnish the body tissues with water thus reducing the amount of toxins that are reabsorbed from the intestines along with the enema water.

Do not forget that the enema should be taken once daily without fail and more often if necessary. Evening is recommended as a good time for the enema because it insures peaceful sleep. The enema will shorten the fast by getting rid of the retained wastes more quickly.

Some people fear that the enema can become habit forming but you will have to want to become addicted to it for this to happen. Even when not fasting a weekly enema is strongly recommended, especially for anyone who continues to eat harmful foods. It is always an aid to cleansing, but it does not compare with the good obtained from entirely avoiding all bad foods.

"And his bowels became full with abominable filthiness, with oozing streams of decay; and multitudes of abominable worms have their habitation there."
(Essene Gospel of Peace)

COLONIC IRRIGATION

In connection with enemas you will often see the term colonic irrigation which is not very well known. The colonic irrigation or "colonic" is a type of super enema and is done by the application of a continuous stream of water into the colon which is intended to fill and flush the colon. This is not a procedure which can be done at home. It requires a special machine and a qualified and licensed operator. It is usually offered by chiropractors, naturopaths, massuers, and an occasional enlightened M.D. The procedure takes from one-half to three-quarters of an hour.

The tube used for the colonic, though like the standard enema tube, is made so that the water flows both in and out. It is equipped with a vacuum pump that sucks out the water and debris. Most discharge lines have a clear tube which allows the operator to see what wastes are being removed from the colon.

The colonic is always valuable and its effects are superior to the standard enema and if available, should be taken every third day, but it is not required in order to fast. When you take a colonic you can skip the enema. Also the person who administers the irrigation is in many cases familiar with fasting and the time it takes to perform the irrigation allows you time for professional consultation about your fast. Colonics range in price from $8 to $25. The colonic is excellent both while detoxifying and during the fast.

"So I tell you truly, suffer the angel of water to baptise you also within, that you may become free from all your past sins, and that within likewise you may become as pure as the river's foam sporting in the sunlight." (Essene Gospel of Peace)

CHAPTER 8

WHILE FASTING

After properly preparing your body's system through detoxification, you should feel comfortable about moving into a water fast. The water fast is the true fast, and so called fasts using fruit juice of one or more kinds are not fasts. They are correctly designated at a mono diet.

As you begin the fast drink only distilled water. If you still feel the need of extra cleansing help or to vary taste, one tablespoon of unprocessed, unheated honey and/or the strained juice of one lemon or lime can be added to a gallon of water. However plain water is the most effective. No liquids, tap water, teas, fruit, vegetable juices or any other mixture is useable.

Do not be hesitant at the idea of living on just water. You are not living on distilled water but rather living off of the excess nutritive substances and fat that the body did not need and stored as fat which now is acting as fuel.

"We have no means of knowing how much of a reserve store of vitamins the body possesses, nor do we know where all these reserves are stored . . . But we may be sure of one thing, namely, that these stores are sufficient to outlast the most prolonged fast. (Dr. Hereward Carrington)

Although many people overlook it, the role and function of water is crucial in the body. Water, like air, has always been taken for granted. Many people are not aware that water constitutes approximately two-thirds of our weight. A person of average size and weight contains about one hundred pounds of water. The gray matter of the brain is eighty-five percent water and more than ninety percent of blood plasma is water.

Water is more than just water. It is also the vehicle for food material absorbed from the digestive canal. It is also the thermostat or regulator of body temperature and is a lubricant for many of the body's moving parts, one of its more mechanical functions. It aids in the movement of joints and in the friction of the intestinal coils against each other.

Water will aid in the softening and dissolving of impacted fecal matter and help in its elimination. Constipation is a condition in which stools are hard and dry and difficult to pass. The less water there is in the intestines, the worse the constipation. This is why juicy fruits and vegetables are used in pre-fast detoxification and not bread and cheese. The fruits and vegetables contain much more fiber and fluids. Water washes out and cleans the stomach and intestines and constitutes, in fact, a sort of second enema.

During fasting you can lose practically all of your stored glycogen and all of your reserves of fat and nearly half of your protein, either that stored or built in to your structure, without any real danger. But a loss of ten percent of body water is serious and a loss of twenty-twenty-five percent means certain death.

Maintenance of your water level is of the utmost importance. During such illnesses as cholera or dysentery, diarrhea will carry water out of the body and doesn't allow the water taken by mouth to be absorbed. These illnesses reduce the volume of blood by reducing its water content. With water loss, blood becomes thicker and causes greater friction increasing the difficulty of circulation. Corpuscles stick in the heart, and it is then no longer able to reach its normal output, blood pressure can drop sharply resulting in shock.

Seldom does such an unnatural loss of water occur. Nevertheless, we naturally lose water continuously. Breathing carries away water which is visible on cold days when it turns to vapor or frosts a window pane. On dry days you can lose up to a pint of water through normal breathing. Water loss through perspiration is well known and is easily a pint a day when body activity is moderate. The main dispeller of water is the kidneys, by which non-violatile wastes are eliminated. During fasting a large quantity of water is essential for proper maintenance and cleansing of the body and its systems. If the body is not supplied with water, it will use its stored supply when wastes are released and must be expelled. This is one cause of frequent urination during fasting. Stored water is also released in order to keep the blood normal. It is interesting to know that during total water deprivation, the heart and brain are the last organs to give up their supply of water protecting the body to the end.

Water drunk in large amounts will not dilute the blood but is deposited in your water bank, which is mainly within the body's connective tissues. Any water not needed is expelled in the normal ways. If the water supply runs low your salivary glands will give up their holdings. The salivary glands release is ninety-eight percent water but even this source will diminish and fail to keep the throat and mouth comfortable if not replenished. The most unpleasant sensation of dryness — "cotton mouth" as it is sometimes called — is a symptom of thirst that will strongly motivate you to replenish the body's water supply.

AVOID FLUORIDATED TAP WATER

The dangers of using tap water — that water provided to the home by the community — is being talked about a lot these days. Rightly so. Almost all tap water is dangerous, containing fluorides and chlorine. Don't let anyone tell you otherwise. Fluoridated tap water should be avoided entirely. Distilled water and filtered rain water that has been warmed directly by the sun's light and rays are best. Distilled water is soft. If you wash your hair in distilled water you will see how soft it is. Distilled water is the purest water on earth and is free of all harmful inorganic substances. If any water that has any minerals whatsoever is used during fasting, autolysis will not take place as effectively as it would if distilled water was drunk as minerals can be considered foods. Any nutrient of the least amount will be attacked for food diverting autolysis from oxidizing fat within the body. Any nutrient at all will also stimulate the stomach into activity and hunger will surely return which makes it easier to go on a complete water fast than a juice fast.

Distilled water is available in one gallon or five gallon containers. It is best to purchase distilled water in the five gallon containers as it is not only cheaper but comes in glass; whereas, the gallon containers are often plastic. Whether buying or storing water, avoid plastic containers because they cannot be sterilized for reuse.

Distilled water should not be left in open containers as it will readily take up impurities from the atmosphere.

Again, during the fasting you may add the juice of one fresh squeezed lemon or lime (for added cleansing) to each gallon and sweeten slightly with a tablespoon of honey to vary the taste.

For an extended fast it is easier and more convenient to prepare you drinking mixture by the gallon. For a gallon of water add the juice of one fresh squeezed lemon or lime and a tablespoon of unprocessed raw (unpasteurized and unfiltered) honey. Anyone suffering from diabetes should use Tupelo honey only, which is also readily available in health food stores. Do not refrigerate. Never shock the body by drinking anything too hot or too cold. Remember, the nearest to body temperature, 98.6, the better. Too cold a drink drops body temperature constricting the intestinal canal. Drink up to a whole gallon everyday that you fast and keep a two quart minimum. In any case drink to satisfy your thirst. More water will be craved during summer than winter. Water should always be drunk when there is thirst, and it is true that a glass or two of water will help offset the hunger sensations in the stomach which occur during the first few days.

ENERGY DURING FASTING

As the fast progresses, the strength of the faster will be found to increase, especially if he is ill at the start of the fast. As all toxins leave the body, energy will return or get stronger. Weakness is related to disease and not often to lack of food.

Also, after the first few days into your fast, your body's previously constant use of energy to digest food comes to a stop. Power that your body would orginarily have used to convert food into energy and body tissue through digestion and assimilation, is now conserved and extended to the rest of the organism. The new use of this energy gives added strength and efficiency for healing and the elimination of toxins.

The response is similar to what happens in an automobile using its air conditioner. When the air conditioner is turned off, the car will increase its speed without increasing the gas supply. The engine receives greater power. During a fast it is not unusual to sleep only two or three hours a night and wake up completely refreshed and energized.

The contrary experience is the fatigue felt after large meals particularly such as the family holiday dinner. We have all seen the older family members go off to sleep all over the living room and even the young ones noticeably slowed down. This is the result of over-eating and so burdening the digestive system with too much work. A great deal more blood must flow to the organs of digestion and a lot more energy is required to move it where it is needed and to then carry away the excess while also digesting as much as possible. This leaves the rest of the body, especially the brain, heart, lungs, and muscles too deprived and fatigued to be active.

It takes a large amount of energy to pass a huge meal through the gastro-intestinal tract, the 28 foot tube that runs from the mouth to the rectum.

The entire nervous, digestive, circulatory, respiratory, and glandular system arrest much of their activity during a fast. The faster's system has been said to resemble that of a hibernating animal. Furthermore, not only physical rest is bestowed on the faster but also psychological rest. Because of the effects to the mind, many people fast in order to achieve spiritual "highs." When the body is truly at rest as during a fast it is most easy to avoid body awareness and so forget its existence, which is an ideal situation for meditation.

SLEEP

Sometimes the faster has difficulty sleeping, is restless and tosses and turns. In this case the faster either needs no sleep, has neglected drinking his water, or has failed to take his enema. This restlessness can be a sign that toxins are being released and are being reabsorbed into the blood stream. Recently, during the supervision of a 21 year old female's fast, on the seventh day she could not sleep because of food dreams. At one time she dreamed of a family dinner that she attended years before. This dream recurred several times during the night and was accompanied by much discomfort. I asked her if she had taken her enema that day and she replied that she had not. She was given a high enema and a brief air bath which restored her rest. The enema removed the wastes which were being reabsorbed from the colon and ended the toxification which caused the problem.

The matter being reabsorbed had probably been in her colon at least as long as the time when the woman had taken the food and that is why she flashed back to those times of her life. Nevertheless, regardless of the cause food dreams are most likely to be remembered and discussed by fasters because of their natural preoccupation with food while they are depriving themselves of.

Because the body operates more efficiently during a fast the amount of sleep required may be reduced, but the rest of other kinds, especially for those undertaking fasts of more than 21 days, and care in the use of your energy must be maintained.

LEARN TO CONSERVE ENERGY

During a long fast any effort wasted in the early part will be felt later. Even when all care is taken, you can sometimes tire easily, so always move cautiously climbing stairs only one at a time and bending and stooping with care. Remember always rise slowly and try to hold onto something. Blood pressure goes down greatly while fasting and changes in elevation can cause extreme dizziness, even fainting (see page 78). Coordination is also affected and it is wise not to drive during the long fast. Driving and all of the routine activities are far more consuming of energy than you think: reading, writing, watching television, listening to radio or music, talking, and especially sex should be avoided while fasting for long periods.

The ideal condition for a long fast is in a place of isolation in nature, but when this is not possible every attempt must be made to maximize your time in the air and sun to avoid all unnecessary contacts with all parts of the world's distractions. Because of the changes which you undergo you may find that you are clumsier than before, so you will want to develop new ways of behavior.

As the long fast continues you will see that fewer and fewer things will stimulate you to overt action. Your methods of walking, bathing, etc. will change. All of your activities will naturally move toward smoothness and ease, any way that is less tiring. The methods you develop for energy utilization will be beneficial when the fast is over also. As a result of fasting your whole tempo will slow and you will live in a more relaxed and healthy way no longer wasting energy unnecessarily. By fasting, chronic nail biters and nervous foot tappers will often break these habits.

Whether fasting for short or long periods of time, your energy will fluctuate. There will be times of weakness. These will be no problem. Rest, conserve and continue to health.

EXERCISE DURING FASTING

Whether fasting or not proper daily exercise plays an essential role in the maintenance of a healthy body and gives the body the relaxation it also needs. Exercise and relaxation in balance permit the body's "intrinsic energy" to flow as it should. A properly balanced body is a security force against disease and the invasion of enervating distractions so prevalent in our busy urban existence. Some of the benefits of exercise are presented in the following list.

- All internal organs improve and increase their functioning.
- Congestions (constipation) of toxins, like cholesterol increased blood flow.
- Weight is redistributed properly, loose flesh is removed and skin is toned.
- Lungs are strengthened and enlarged which speeds the delivery of oxygen in larger amounts to all cells and removes more waste matter.
- The muscles along the digestive tract are toned and strengthened helping to cure "potbelly" or what is often prematurely thought to be "middle age spread."
- Circulation is improved allowing more flow of blood wherever needed, especially the heart.
- The entire body is purified and the increased blood flow benefits the brain, producing greater mental energy and alertness.
- The entire system is revitalized, stimulated and refreshed.
- Digestion is benefitted and constipation is eliminated.

TYPES OF EXERCISE

Exercise is as important for the faster as for anyone, but he must be careful to employ those kinds of exercise which do not debilitate — remember that you are fasting, not body building. The following types of exercise are nearly effortless if performed correctly. They are walking, Hatha Yoga, and Tai Chi. Hatha Yoga and Tai Chi also offer the further benefit of peace of mind, control over the senses, mastery of the lower self, and the ability to experience the Divine Grace that powers life itself.

Walking

Walking is good during both the short and long fast. Three to ten miles are not too far to walk daily during a short fast. Those fasting beyond 21 days should moderate their distance in order to have the exercise be beneficial and not enervating. Fasters need exercise but they need to conserve energy also.

Try to find a natural setting in which to take your walk. Avoid places where you have to always be on guard against traffic both of cars and people. Merely having to be aware of traffic causes a drain of energy needed for your maintenance of a comfortable balance. If possible, walk in the woods or the park. In these settings you encounter the kind, soothing effects of mother nature. Walk easily and relaxed; enjoy it all confident that nature is enjoying you in your newly recovered relationship with her. Walking repetitiously the same route over and over is not good as, for example, repeatedly walking around the block. Through the park or in the woods would be better as they offer a constant change. Repetition such as swimming laps in the pool or weight lifting is even more detrimental to the constant unobstructed flow of energy which we all need in order to maintain internal harmony.

Hatha Yoga

Hatha Yoga is an Eastern system of exercises, that is an ideal method for maintaining a proper balance of the body and the mind. It is a psycho-physical method of exercises based upon thousands of years of old profound knowledge of the inter-action of the mind-body.

Lost health can be restored and with it increased mind strength that leads to the realization of the power of your spirit which has for so long merely been waiting for you to discover it.

Hatha Yoga is made up of a series of postures (asanas) which are to be achieved without strain and held comfortably.

During these slow, smooth motions, the body is in a state of efficiency. They are performed along with controlled deep breathing which oxygenates the blood and cleanses it. Energy is thus accumulated rather than expended in these exercises. It is effortless when done correctly.

The entire body system benefits by the postures. The bending and twisting positions put pressure on the endocrine glands, balancing out their functions and thus improving all systems, including the digestive and eliminative functions, as well as the rebuilding processes. The postures relax and tone the muscles and the nervous system, loosen joints, stretch ligaments, stimulate circulation, aid in digestion, and gently massage the internal organs.

Totally, the aim of the postures is a controlled body and mind free from all unnecessary disturbances, much the same as one of fasting's goals, cleaning and maintaining the body which is recognized as the dwelling of God. When such a condition of balance and cleanliness is reached you can discover your true self, your Divine self. Once the postures become steady and the breathing controlled, the mind, which St. Teresa called "that uncontrollable animal," and which can be our worst enemy, begins to be less of a distraction and frees a new life energy, the energy of peace and perfection.

For those not familiar with yogic techniques, there are many books designed for self teaching; and in many cities, there are instructors who give inexpensive courses.

Tai Chi

Tai Chi (Supreme Ultimate) is a Chinese martial art that is nevertheless, soft, smooth, and effortless. In fact, it replenishes the system through relaxation so that the forces which the Chinese refer to as Yin-Yang can restore themselves and return to a proper balance. Tai Chi is not only effective as an exercise, and self-defense, but is also an excellent form of meditation.

After studying and performing Tai Chi for many years, I found it to be tremendously effective in retaining or regaining energy during fasting.

In Tai Chi all movement comes from the Tian Tien located about one and a half inches below the navel. The Chi energy

(Japanese call it Ki) powers every movement. With practice you discover that effort and strength are unnecessary; in fact, they are obstructions to the use of Chi, a natural force of nature.

Tai Chi gives you everything when you do nothing. Done correctly, Tai Chi is effortless. For its proper doing three things are essential. (1) Correct instruction. Make sure that your teacher stresses total relaxation. (2) Preseverance. Only through your own practice will you come to an understanding of the principle. (3) Natural ability. Your ability to follow the principle of effortlessness is basic. Sick and older people often learn more quickly as they are less caught by the notion of strength.

Once again, remember you are fasting and not building the muscles. You are resting and cleansing and should not attempt to do other than effortless exercise. Rejuvenative exercise is very important. Use all caution not to deplete your energy. Enervation is a cause of sickness.

SUNBATHING

The sun, the source of all earthly life can be considered lunch for the faster. People are light dependent beings composed of "billions of worlds", each like the earth called cells. Without the sun's essential cosmic power, all earthly living things would cease to exist. Sunlight is essential to all animal life and plants for the process of assimilating, or nourishing themselves from the atmosphere and soil. All life bends toward the sun, and total exclusion of sunlight results in the death of plants and may cause several health problems in people.

Daily exposure to the sun's rays aids the human organism in the performance of all its functions, acts as a healer, and will help any skin condition, itching or scaling to quickly improve itself. Sunlight also aids in elimination and the absorption of oxygen through the skin, and creates, by the action of light on skin cells, or by the action of ultraviolet rays on a variety of substances, a supply of vitamin D which is essential in maintaining a balanced body chemistry.

Many authorities have said that the long term effect of fresh air and sunlight is more important to a longer, healthier, life than actual diet itself.

Fasting or not, daily sunbathing offers a power of unlimited strength which you may tap. The best method is to use a private, natural setting and remove all your clothes for at least half an hour every day. If you don't live where this total exposure is permissible, you can build a small enclosure very easily and inexpensively in your back yard or on your roof or terrace to protect you from scandal and the police.

Let the sun soothe and embrace your entire body. This pleasing warmth will enable the tense individual to relax relieving all stress and nervousness from the body, unless the sunning is overdone. Although sunbathing is highly beneficial, the sun is potentially dangerous. Avoid the rays of the direct sun from ten a.m. until two p.m. or later in the summer when the sun is at its hottest. Early morning or late afternoon is best. Gradually build up to one-half hour, starting with five to fifteen minutes the first day and adding five minutes each day. Always avoid prolonged sunbathing whether you are fasting or not. Lengthy exposure destroys skin and body cells. Keep in mind that when using white sheets or blankets or sunning on white sand beaches, the sun is reflected and becomes stronger.

While sunbathing use your olive or almond oil to prevent dehydration and to aid in beautifying the skin. After a little use of a good natural oil you will learn how readily the skin absorbs it without leaving any odor but only a bright glow. Try to sunbathe close to home. Driving or riding back and forth can drain you of energy on a long fast.

It is better, but not necessary, if you can sunbathe away

from the city taking into consideration that pollutants in the air act as filters drastically changing the quality of sunlight. Avoid artificial tanning lotions, creams and oils. Avoid also simulated sun source lamps. Remember the *Sun is King* and should be highly respected and received in its purest possible form.

AIR BATHING

Like the sun, our air is also taken much for granted. There is much pure air in the sky above, but not much is found today at ground level where man lives. As long as windy turbulence mixes the dirty ground air with the pure supply above, we can survive. Since pollutants are much heavier than air, higher altitudes (mountains) offer more sun and cleaner air to the faster.

To exist, man must breathe. Cut off his oxygen supply even briefly and man dies. It is easy to see how basic and simple is his need for pure air. Everything your body breathes influences the body. This influence may be nutritious or poisonous. Today all air is polluted. Some areas are more polluted than others. All we can do is adapt to this pollution and take measures to prevent it from becoming worse and eliminate the source of already existing causes.

Not only do people inhale polluted air from their environment, but some further the internal pollution of their bodies through tobacco smoking. Studies made by Clarence A. Mills, M.D., professor of Experimental Medicine of the University of Cincinnati, and others have led to a general acceptance of the fact that the hazards of tobacco smoking and of general air pollution are, in many respects, almost identical. They also each add to the dangers of the other. Dr. Mills adds,

"If you must smoke, then you'd better live in cleaner air and avoid the urban motor traffic." Or, "If you must live in dirty air and drive in city traffic, then you'd better not smoke."

It is really hard to curtail a tobacco habit, or to quit, when the tobacco industry's advertisers cleverly spend millions yearly on cigarette sales promotion. A sizeable portion of the industry's sales is made to teenagers. It is truly sad when American permits the destruction of our youth by such money greedy people.

If you are going to fast, DON'T SMOKE! If you continue to smoke tobacco during fasting you are further adding toxins to the system at the time when you are trying to remove them. Why try to build up your health through fasting and at the same time tear it back down by smoking? By smoking you are doing yourself even more harm during fasting since the body needs all the fresh air it can get to help in the cleaning and eliminating process. Fasting is a most effective way to give up smoking. Often, after a few weeks of fasting, all desire for tobacco leaves. Many people have conquered the habit through fasting.

Fresh air is vital to every cell in our bodies. As oxygen is breathed, it is carried by the blood to the lungs where the life giving air is exchanged for deadly carbon dioxide. As air enters the lungs, deadly poisonous toxins are released as carbon dioxide is expelled.

Fresh air is essential in the purifying process of the body, while fasting and at all times. Without a good supply of fresh air, the general health standard is lowered and the ground work is laid for the evolution of toxemia, seen most frequently as pneumonia, T.B., bronchitis, sinusitis, emphysema, influenza, and associated heart disease. Lack of fresh air caused by too much indoor living and working, bad ventilation, lack of exercise, too tight and too much clothing, especially in winter

60

time, all aid in lowering the body's resistance to these ills.

Sleep with the windows open, discontinue the breathing of dead recycled air caused by your air conditioning systems. Turn if off forever or run it with the windows open. This is another pitfall of hospitals. Air conditioning or heat is used 365 days a year in most hospitals, while patients gasp for fresh air. A little of nature's fresh air in many cases could have prevented the use of the oxygen mask.

There are many spas and resorts where one can go and fast in a natural setting away from the cities and where sun and air bathing in the nude is permitted. If you haven't the money for a spa, you can drive or hike to the country taking along with you in your pack some books, a sleeping bag and an enema kit.

"Seek the fresh air of the forest and of the fields, and there in the midst of them shall you find the angel of air. Put off your shoes and your clothing and suffer the angel of air to embrace your body: Then breathe long and deeply, that the angel of air may be brought within you. I tell you truly, the angel of air shall cast out of your body all uncleannesses which defiled it without and within." (Essene Gospel of Peace)

Remember that a single tree produces a great deal of pure oxygen. So a forest of trees means an abundance of clean air. A friend of mine, Gordon Brooks, who ran across the U.S. in 1969 and captured the Guiness Book of World Records Title, and then ran once again across the U.S. in 1976 with Dick Gregory on Gregory's bicentennial food run, said that by just running close to bushes or trees he experienced a rush of fresh air and easier breathing.

Fresh air during fasting is highly beneficial to the efficiency of the body to clean itself and the faster should get as much as possible. One should take at least one or two air baths daily while fasting. These can be done in conjunction with the sun bath. Remove all your clothes if possible and feel the air embrace your body. Lets its soothing touch massage your entire body. Move about as if you were swimming in air because you are. Since air is a God given right, don't conceal and shield yourself from its life giving energy.

Practice deep breathing exercises two or three times daily. Breathe through the nose always unless your nasal passages are blocked. If this is the case, such a condition is very quickly relieved by fasting.

While fasting, it is always better to get away from cities and urban traffic by going to the country, mountains, or ocean where the air is cleaner. However, if this is not possible, many benefits are also bestowed on the city faster. It is always better to fast where you are than to allow your system to go on being polluted from within or to allow a disease condition to become worse by putting off a fast.

BODILY CARE

The body is the most precious of all the material creations in the universe. Until it dies, it is the home of the soul. Thus the body deserves great attention and respect.

Regular bathing of the body with pride should be practiced by everyone. Nevertheless, many of us neglect this practice. Often it has been said that people respect their cars and wash them more often than they do their own bodies.

While on a long fast there is more need to wash the body because so much filth and poisons are excreted and passed out through the ninety-six million pores of the skin in the form of moisture and sweat. The skin receives a third of all the blood circulating in the body so a poisonous blood supply means a body surface coated by toxins.

There are also two to three million sweat glands throughout the body found in dense clusters in the feet, hands, armpits, and forehead. These allow perspiration to transport more toxins and further add to the skin's burden during fasting.

During fasting bathing is recommended twice a day and once is a requirement. There is no question here of danger in any acute sense, but without daily bathing the full effect of the fast is not as likely to be obtained because when the toxins are not removed the body will reabsorb them. The bath should always be taken with both pleasure and caution. If the faster is experiencing weakness at bath time, a sponge bath can suffice. If the aid of a friend is obtainable, ask the friend to help you.

Baths should be of short duration. People who like to bathe or shower for long periods of time should discontinue this habit for the period of the fast. Long baths will deplete and enervate the body when energy conservation should be used in every way possible. Do not use extremely hot or cold water. They sap a great deal of energy and may shock the nervous system. The bath should be as close to body temperature as possible, 100° or 38° C.

The entire surface of the body should be scrubbed giving special attention to the perspiration points mentioned earlier. Excellent results are obtained by scrubbing with a Loofa — a sponge — which is available in the health food stores and in many souvenir shops. Scrub with the sponge and a natural soap, one free of animal products or other film and residue depositing agents. Most commercial soaps will coat and often irritate the skin and can contribute to toxification; however there are a few commercially available soaps that are natural and leave no animal residue on the skin. While scrubbing, massage in circles to promote better circulation of the blood.

Rinse then repeat the same process, but this time use only fresh clean water. If you are using a tub bath, release the water and rinse by pouring water over yourself or get under the shower. This will insure that all the secreted toxins will be cleared from the skin. If you were tubbing, it is interesting to take a look at the ring around the tub as the water drains. This will usually give clear evidence that cleansing is taking place.

After the bath, dry yourself well, stay warm, and apply oil to the skin. The oil prevents dehydration of the skin and will make the body smooth and beautiful.

Those troubled by dandruff and flaky scalp often find that these problems disappear as the fast continues. The cause of dandruff like most health problems is traced to toxemia and results from the body's efforts to rid itself of the internal toxins or wastes causing it. Wash the scalp thoroughly with a natural Ph balance shampoo, also available widely and at health stores. Massage the scalp in circles to loosen the scales and to stimulate the circulation, and you will come away feeling tinglingly refreshed.

CARE OF THE MOUTH

The mouth is also an eliminator of toxins during fasting. Breath becomes foul as it expels toxic fumes. (See page 73.) The tongue becomes coated white, probably from the trapping of the more solid particles as when we find our clothes dirtied by atmospheric pollution. From this same matter the teeth often become gummy. To clear these symptoms brush several times a day and brush the tongue. Do not use the commercial toothpastes and powders as they are artificially colored and flavored, and especially don't eat the toothpaste. As the fast progresses all of these symptoms decrease and finally disappear. When they are all gone, it signifies the end or nearly the end of the fast.

THE SAUNA

Anyone suffering from high blood pressure or heart condition should consult a physician before taking a sauna bath.

Uses

- Sauna aids in weight control.
- Sauna quiets nerves and promotes restful sleep.
- Sauna smooths lines of tension from the face.
- Sauna deep cleans the pores leaving skin radiant.
- Sauna stimulates circulation.
- Sauna regulates the body.
- Sauna relaxes over exerted, cramped and tired muscles.
- Sauna gives palliative relief from rheumatism, arthritis, and related ailments.

The sauna is a dry heat bath widely used in the north of Europe, particularly Sweden. It causes profuse sweating which is an effective cleansing for the body inside and out, bathing every pore. Nevertheless, while fasting do not let the heat exceed 130 degrees nor stay in for more than five to ten minutes and do no steaming. Even five minutes will open the skin and dilate the blood vessesl sending the blood rapdily to the surface and expelling toxic wastes through the pores. After the sauna do not shock the body with cold water, as the Swedes do. The faster must always guard against chill. Rinse with warm water but do not overdo this part either. Too much of anything is enervating for the faster's system.

CHAPTER 9

COMMON REACTIONS DURING FASTING

AUTOLYSIS

The cleansing that occurs after food has been withheld for sometime is different from the kind that occurs during pre-fast detoxification. Once the food in the body has been cleared, the fast enters its true health cleansing during which it nourishes itself from within. At this stage the body utilizes its stored nutrients, and all tissue components, even to the cellular level, which are defective in any way. They are consumed. As mentioned earlier, this process of self consumption is called "autolysis." It is the oxidizing of any and all unneeded internal materials. What is least essential to the body is used or oxidized first for food (e.g., diseased cells or tissues, fat and mucus and often tumors).

The more inferior the tissues are, the less hesitation there is about burning them. Gradually, after the deposits of impurities and fat have been consumed, a kind of chiseling work then starts. Every place where there are substances that still need burning, the inner mechanism carries out the work of what Otto Buchinger, M.D. once called,

"A surgeon operating without a knife."

Autolysis is a mechanism by which the faster maintains both life and health. Autolysis both nourishes the body during fasting and in the process releases and eliminates toxins stored in the tissues that would otherwise lead to ill health. During a fast toxins are also released by the mechanical process of tissue contraction that forces mucus and poisons into the blood stream, making them readily available for elimination. When food is removed, the entire body is free to adjust to the needs of cells and tissues which in turn adjust to cleanse themselves, a level of self-care not achievable by any other method than fasting.

All released toxic wastes are then carried away by the blood stream and the lymph system, using the bowels, kidneys, eyes, ears, nose and skin, (actually the entire body) as the outlets of elimination for the dislodged wastes. All toxic wastes that leave the body represent more weight leaving the body.

It is during the first few days of your fast that you discover that your previous way of eating will effect you in proportion to how badly and how much you were in the habit of eating, especially junk food — all the heavy breads, cakes, confections and candies and, of course, meat, drugs and alcohol. Many fasting attempts have failed because of ignorance of the nature of the opening days of the fast when if any real difficulty is to be encountered it will occur. During this period of the fast all at once you release various obstructions of your body's plumbing system into the blood stream in the form again of mucus and toxins. When this release is rapid and elimination does not occur you can often be made to feel ill. And though too dramatic a name in most cases, this is what is called the "crisis period."

This feeling of illness is almost always slight but in most cases it is thought to be a reason for breaking the fast and that it must be that food is needed. This is a self-fulfilling diagnosis since when the fast is broken and eating is resumed nutrients are again obtained from this food, autolysis is stopped and the rumblings and contractions of organs and tissues also ends. Toxins are no longer released and those in the blood are either reabsorbed or eliminated causing all symptoms of the so-called "crisis" to disappear; but, in fact, actually the toxins are now poisoning the body in a truly dangerous way. The release of toxins is why many people get weak, have headache, and feel miserable if they don't eat on time. The truth is that the more waste that people collect in their systems, the more food they must eat in order to stop the elimination that occurs. Thus the healthiest seeming people sometimes have to pass through what seems a stage of illness (really only the discomfort of cleansing) to get to a higher level of health. There is nothing to fear. The crisis is a paper tiger even when it occurs, which is seldom and then usually it is very mild. If there is any difficulty, maintain your faith and tranquility and the problem will soon disappear. A little discomfort now will stop more severe pain later in your life. Sooner or later everyone must die but while we are here in these bodies we can at least live our lives in the best physical way possible, in health and happiness.

Usually the second fast is easier in the beginning than the first was. The bowels and the whole system are usually not so corrupt as they had been during the first fast. You will not experience the weakening effect of the poisons in the system to such a degree as in the initial fast.

When fasting there are several common reactions that may be anticipated. None are cause for alarm and should give no reason or excuse for ending a fast. Remember once again, the degree of discomfort you will have during the first few days will be decided by how well you prepared for the fast and how well your colon was washed out by the use of the enema and colonic irrigations before and during the fast.

Headache and Weakness

As mentioned earlier, when most people skip a meal or a day of eating, one of the first things that happen is the appearance of a headache usually accompanied by weakness. Because food is cut off the system looks elsewhere for its nutrients. As the body consumes its own stores, the process of autolysis is quickly in full effect. Because fat is being burned, lodged poisons are released and enter your blood stream and find their way to the brain, causing self-poisoning (auto-intoxication).

As autolysis occurs the entire system gets weak and you experience a slight but consistent headache. This sort of problem usually continues until these poisonous wastes pass out through the organs of elimination, or until food is introduced back into the body. As food is once again consumed, autolysis stops, and the body turns back again to the new food stuffs for its nutrients. No more fasting, no more headache and weakness, because toxins stop entering the blood. This is why when the toxic person misses a meal or two and gets a bit poisoned, it feels so alleviating when he eats once again; he swears up and down that this ill feeling was because of a lack of food. However, if people would learn that his freeing of stored toxic matter started by missing a meal or two that causes these symptoms and not the need for food, they would then be able to see that these wastes are corrupting their health and would soon realize how badly fasting is needed. Headache and weakness or other symptoms will also be felt by anyone who has conditioned his system to the regular use of stimulants like coffee, tea, beer, wine, stronger alcohol, or drugs. When these stimulants are removed from nerves and cells there is, almost of necessity, a withdrawal reaction. But the person so accustomed (all of us almost) can keep in mind that fasting will break the stimulant habit by clearing away the provocation to it with the residues it has deposited even in the cells. Scientific fasting washes them out and flushes them away.

Be aware that headache and weakness do not usually occur or are very slight if pre-fast detoxification is carried out properly. However, if discomfort does arise in the beginning, don't quit; for it usually disappears in three days as the body adjusts itself to fasting.

The process of fasting itself causes some of the discomfort because the gas formed from decomposing cells or poisonous excrements still remaining in the bowels may be reabsorbed and so add to the stuff which must enter the system before it can be removed. Oxidizing cells become toxic waste like any other but it is fasting and only fasting that has the power to both clean and renew the system to the cellular level. All cells that contain toxins are, in a manner of speaking, either squeezed clean or destroyed and replaced.

Nevertheless, no matter what causes the symptoms, with proper care they are usually quite mild and are always temporary. All toxic matter is continually being carried away by the entire body. Stick to your water and your enemas and or colonics. Detoxify first and all will be well.

Remember with the proper "drying out," most fasters will experience at most a mild crisis during the first few days of the fast, if any at all.

The first few days if difficult are so because toxins are leaving the body more rapidly than later on in the fast when you become cleaner. As the fast progresses strength will accommodate cleanliness. It is not at all uncommon to feel stronger on the twenty-first day of fasting than on the first or second day, or amazingly enough, to feel better than when you were eating.

But if you do not feel strong and vigorous at any time during your scheduled fast, this is almost never a sign of danger. Energy may be very low off and on throughout a long fast, especially if you have to participate in any other activity at the same time. Remember to conserve energy always, but especially so if you are working while fasting. Do only what you have to do and remember that your energy will fluctuate.

Loss of Weight

It has been thoroughly demonstrated that almost all who have mistreated their bodies to the point of becoming obese (obesity — which is defined as being 20 percent over one's normal weight), have colons that are impacted (some packed almost to closure) with as much as thirty five pounds of decaying fecal matter. Most adults who are accustomed to the American diet carry around with them between five and fifteen pounds of this colonic obstruction. By using the enema and colonics during the fast, this colonic matter is broken up and washed out of the intestines. Cleaning the colon flattens the stomach and lightens the body — weight loss is a very supportive visible result for the overweight faster.

Most fasters lose between two and three pounds during the first twenty four hours when the previous meals are removed from the bowels. Also during the beginning state of the fast the body loses its accumulated water. In some cases obese people have lost up to twenty pounds during a week long fast and up to ten pounds in just a weekend.

Weight loss is the most obvious outward result of fasting.

If you fail to take your daily enema, you can expect that the degree of loss of weight is apt to be less than usual that day.

After a week to ten days of fasting you will probably reduce the amount of weight lost each day because the water that left the body in the beginning, is now reduced. At this time you will lose weight in proportion to the amount of fat stored on your body. This is a much slower process than in the beginning, usually a pound per day.

By becoming thinner you can live longer. As mentioned before, man is mostly water. A one-hundred sixty pound man is one hundred pounds of water. As soon as you stop eating, large amounts of water are expelled from the body. The water's bulk and that of the eliminated solid wastes, plus the oxidized fat produces a quick and substantial drop in weight. An interesting side effect is when you have to buy your bathing suit in the boys' or girls' department.

During a water fast there is no counting of calories as in most diets, just the counting of reduced pounds. Americans spend millions of dollars yearly to get rid of unwanted pounds when the most effective and natural cure for obestity is free.

Fat is profit for many doctors and all pharmaceutical companies. By using diet plans and pills people may lose a few pounds but they usually gain the weight back in no time. Fasting, on the other hand, breaks many food addictions and teaches self-discipline. In many cases, for the first time the faster will have enough self control to stay slim. During your fast weigh yourself each day. Record the amount of lost pounds for comparison to other diets.

Foul Breath

One of the earliest signs that a fast has begun is foul breath. This is a sign of a foul digestive tract and the cause of this odor is all the toxic matter which the fast causes to be eliminated via the mucus membranes of the mouth. An early sign of the coming end of a fast is when the breath becomes sweet again. This may occur before the actual need to stop the fast. It may, therefore, not be a sure sign but an alert. Another possible source of the odor may be impacted fecal matter and sluggish or reduced bowel action. The noxious gas from the fermentation in the bowels of this residue can reach the lungs by osmosis and is then discharged by the breath.

Heavily Coated Tongue

Whether sick or healthy everyone deposits a sticky, white greyish mucus on the tonuge once the first day of total fasting (twenty four hours) has been achieved. The tongue will be coated in proportion to the impurities in the body.

The same excretions causing the bad odor of the breath are also the cause of the mucus that coats the tongue. However, these excretions come primarily from the lungs and are a sure sign of elimination and true fasting. The tongue also is an organ of elimination and an excellent barometer of the fast. When the tongue clears it is almost surely a sign that the fast is ended. Beyond this point there is danger of starving.

The coating can be removed from the tongue and should be for comfort two or three times a day simply by brushing the tongue when you are brushing your teeth. Don't be too brisk and irritate your tongue, but brush it. As long as the coating remains you can be sure that your system is being nourished, and you need have no fear of doing yourself harm by starving or deficiency disease like protein (amino acid) deprivation or vitamin reduction.

Remain calm and the body will care for you and itself. Interfere with it as little as possible and all will be well.

Chilling

During a fast the body's resistance to cold is lowered and keeping warm becomes a major concern. The feet especially become prone to chilling. This is why fasting during the warm seasons or going to a warm climate is preferred and recommended. However, people have fasted in the midst of winter and have kept sufficiently warm with the use of artificial heat and warm clothes.

By keeping warm your body will conserve energy and permit more rapid elimination; whereas chilling will retard elimination and waste energy, and could lead to the urge to end you fast.

Frequent Urination

As a fast progresses water is eliminated in order to act as a vehicle to carry released impurities out of the body. Recall that while fasting the entire body functions to remove wastes, but, of course, in the case of water the kidneys play the major role. The frequency of urination increases because all liquids taken in quickly picks up toxins which the body wants to rid itself of. Furthermore, the kidneys will also absorb water from the tissues and the colon especially during and after enemas. The body turns everything to efficient cleansing and weight loss when fasting.

Dark Clouded Urine

At the start of the fast, the urine becomes dark and clouded, and strongly acid. This is caused by dissolved uric acid, phosphates, bile pigments, and mucus.

As the fast progresses, the color of the urine will become light and cleaner. Next to the colon, the kidneys carry the biggest job in removing waste from the body.

On your fast you can personally witness cleaning taking place by urinating into a test tube. Let the urine filled test tube stand for twenty-four to thirty-six hours then examine the sediment at the bottom of the tube. As you become cleaner, the sediment decreases. Some fasters will expel sand and gravel from the urinary tract. In most cases, however, this grit is not large enough to create pain or difficulty while urinating. However, in some cases, pain in the form of a burning sensation is experienced. This pain is caused by the releasing of sand and gravel from disintegrating stones resulting from abnormal secretions of the liver, kidneys, and gall bladder. These abnormal secretions are responsible for the precipitation of the mineral elements of these secretions and the bringing forth of stones. These deposits may form in the gall bladder, or in the liver and kidneys. Stones are caused by an unhealthy life style. During a fast, sand and gravel will perhaps be passed by many people even without large stones. Often large stones of the liver, kidneys, and gall bladder disintegrate and pass out by fasting without the use of a surgeon's knife.

Dark, Foul Stools

As I have mentioned before, the average person's colon can be impacted with as much as ten to thirty-five pounds of decayed feces. Hardened bowel wastes of unelimated stool may have been glued to the walls and pockets of the colon since childhood. It is difficult to imagine what decomposed food matter must be like after storage at almost 100 degrees for many years. It will not remain a matter of imagination. You will distinguish this rotted mucus laden stool by its bad odor and its dark color, dark brown to black (normal color of stool is a light tan or the color of foods previously eaten).

During a fast these impactions gradually loosen and with the aid of enemas and colonics are washed from the body because no food is being ingested to block its dissolution. I was amazed that on the thirty-fifth day of total fasting I was still passing foul stools daily. But then on the thirty-eighth day the enema water flowed out of my bowels as clear and clean as it went in.

In rare cases of fasting, people have eliminated along with their stool, worms. When you see worms wiggle in the toilet basin, you will then realize that your previous diet was corrupt and unnatural. This startling evidence will usually change the entire diet pattern of an individual, in turn his entire life will change also.

Body Odor

When fasting perspiration smells bad because it is also carrying the disease causing toxins: drugs, particles of uric acid (largely from meat consumption), decomposed cells, and other matter out of the body. All of which gives a good indication of your true health and bodily condition. You will see, smell, and taste cleansing taking place. What you will be aware of as to badness of taste, smell, or appearance will depend on your own internal condition which is dependent on your dietary habits over the years. The combination of foul breath and unpleasant body odor makes it advisable to keep your distance from other people. When the cleansing process is at its height no deodorant is capable of covering the odor. Most artificial deodorants are not safe and should not be used whether fasting or not. People whose diets are clean with pure and natural foods do not need to use deodorants anyway.

Also, do not forget that the daily changing of clothes is very important because large amounts of toxic excretions get deposited in your clothes making them odorous.

After you have successfully completed your fast, you will realize that you have no need for deodorants. The fast will have removed the cause of the odor leaving none that needs to be concealed. When in good health both body and breath odors should be pleasant, light fragrances and are as long as you maintain a healthful diet of whole, primarily raw foods.

It is truly a pleasure to work all day and still smell clean.

Lowered Blood Pressure

The entire body rests during fasting. Its tempo is much slower than usual after it adjusts to the cutting off of the need for digestion and to maintaining itself by autolysis. The heart slows down and with it circulation which causes a dramatic decrease in blood pressure. Anyone with raised blood pressured will soon realize that fasting is the superior treatment for this problem.

Toxicodermatitis (Skin Eruptions)

When a person is highly toxic, stored up poisons and mucus are eliminated by the body through the pores of the skin in excess sometimes causing skin eruptions. These occasions are rare and announce themselves in the form of open sores, boils, rashes and more commonly facial as well as body acne.

I know of many cases of young people fasting to clear their acne problem and succeeding. One case was a boy late in his teens who fasted because someone had told him that his facial acne problem would be corrected. After much disappointment and wasted money spent on creams, soaps, pads and cover-up lotions, he was willing to try anything and decided to start a seven day fast. The first few days of his total fast his condition became slightly worse, (this was the result of cleansing and more toxins than usual were surfacing.) Then on the third day of the fast, his pimples began to disappear. On the seventh day of the fast, he was convinced that he had finally found a sure cure and was overjoyed to look in the mirror and see a fair complexion on the way.

Larger skin eruptions, boils, etc, are very rare. Out of one hundred twenty people who fasted with Dick Gregory for 7 days during the Christmas holiday of 1975 at Dr. Ralph Abernathy's Baptist Church in Atlanta, only one person suffered boils, and only two suffered rashes. This 7 day fast was held in order to bring attention to the food shortage in America. The fast was supported by such celebrities as Muhammad Ali, John and Yoko Lennon, Cesar Chavez, Stevie Wonder, Eugene McCarthy, Barbra Streisand, Andrew Young, and Richard Dreyfuss. With all of the problems in America today, we cannot ignore the possibility of a "food shortage." The 120 participants of Mr. Gregory's fast learned not only how to fast but were rewarded with the blessing that if there ever was a food shortage and people were forced to go without food, that they could both physically and psychologically outlast the crisis because of their newly acquired knowledge of fasting.

Irritability

If you spent most of your life eating and being conditioned by "tasty" divitalized foods, as we all have, it is really hard to realize how comfortable sitting in Mother Nature's lap can be. However, just the initial desire to fast is a good sign that you want to help yourself to a better, healthier and happier tomorrow. But you must be willing to break and give up the old habits of eating junk foods that are no good for the body and mind or soul. One can only benefit from fasting if he takes fasting seriously and sincerely wants to fast.

The fast can be looked upon as a transition period that falls in between bad and good eating habits. This transition period often seems to be more difficult mentally than physically, leaving the faster both a little confused and irritable, however, both body and mind are responsible.

Again, I refer to the drug or alcohol addict. Take away an addict's stimulant, and he gets irritable. Take away food from a person, he too becomes irritable as food is also considered a stimulant.

Another cause of irritability is stated in the "Synopsis on Nutrition and Behavior" by an anonymous researcher. "A fundamental response of protoplasm is an increase in irritability as a consequence of the gradual depletion of nutritive stores and a decrease in irritability with the replenishment of the stores." This discovery indicates irritability occurs not only in fasting people but also in undernourished people as well. Many mental problems as well as physical problems are caused by improper diets.

The persistent contraction of the digestive organs also reminds the faster of the "hunger sensation." This becomes quite a distraction during the first few days of the fast but diminishes quickly as the fast proceeds.

In addition, there is a slight but consistent increase in auditory acuity, sharpness of hearing, while fasting. Increased irritability can be indirectly traced to the fact that simple sounds and noises are disturbing and bothersome to the faster and a direct physiological basis in the heightened auditory sensitivity. Along with hearing, touch, smell and tastes are also rendered more acute.

Aggravation is why you should fast alone. Go to the country, and pick a good climate. Good weather definitely will boost the spirits of the faster. Once during a long fast I went from north Florida's cold winter season to the tropics of the Island of Key West on the twenty-first day of a forty day fast and experienced an overwhelming amount of joy and happiness because of the simple pleasant surroundings.

So make things easy for yourself, tell your companions, if you must, that you might experience irritability during your fast and for them to have compassion for you. They should understand rather than become irritable also.

Try to avoid all persons who do not understand fasting. The best rule is to tell no one of your fast. Do not "set yourself up" by dealing with people who are totally in a different frame of mind than you, for you are experiencing a totally new view on life than ever before, and as you adapt to this new life you will soon recognize that your life style of yesterday was probably the cause of both your physical and spiritual suffering.

> "That thou appear not unto men to fast, but unto thy Father which is in secret: And thy Father, which seeth in secret, shall reward thee openly." (St. Matthew 6-18)

As you make the transition and finish your fast, you will become a new person, in most cases much better off than before. It is much like the blind person who has had an operation in order to regain sight. On the "big" day of removing the bandages, he for the first time, sees. So will the faster also see a life new to his eyes as he experiences a "rebirth" and becomes "enlightened" in many ways. Jesus not only gave sight to the physically blind, but the spiritually blind as well. The word light in enlightened goes further than words can ever describe.

During times of irritability have patience. Go for a walk, meditate or just do what you feel you must and soon the irritable feeling will pass as all things must pass.

Often the irritable feeling will occur around the time that you normally eat breakfast, lunch, or dinner. If this is the case, a glass of water, a book, or any hobby should be employed as a distraction from the idea of eating.

STAND UP SLOWLY

As mentioned earlier, blood pressure lowers, the amount of time it takes for blood to reach the brain is reduced so dizziness easily occurs with any quick change of elevation. Never get up rapidly whether lying or sitting down. The blood will not move as quickly as the body. The deprived brain will cause great dizziness or even a black out. Arise slowly, hold on to something, and stretch like a cat. Avoid all abrupt movements like jumping up to answer the phone or to answer the doorbell.

Fainting is very rare but it can occur so be careful of your movements and share in the rest which your inner body is enjoying.

NAUSEA

Because of the recirculation of toxins in the system, a nauseous feeling is no surprise.

Nausea, accompanied by vomiting is rare but does occur in some cases and can become very annoying. As soon as either or both of these discomforts cease, the real comfort and pleasures of fasting return. The faster will at this time feel much better than before the symptoms developed. These symptoms are only a sign that a higher stage of health has been achieved.

FEVER

The healthy individual who does not overeat and has eaten

naturally previous to fasting, will in most cases have no change in his temperature during the fast. Fever comes from the presence of toxemia.

It is those who previous to the fast, have been wrongly fed bad food or too much, develop a fever during fasting. Elimination proceeds at a rapid rate and toxic material is put into the bloodstream. There is no need for alarm. In most cases fever, if it occurs, is temporary.

CHAPTER 10

WHEN TO BREAK THE FAST

As I mentioned throughout the book, there are several signals that tell the faster when to end the fast. These indications however, do not apply to the faster who has predetermined the time that he will end his fast, for one cannot in most cases tell when the natural end of the cleansing fast will occur.

These signs only occur when one has fasted to the time when the body has eliminated and cleansed out all impurities. However, in some circumstances, there are adverse signals telling the faster to end the cleansing fast early. This is why consultation with a specialist throughout the long fast is recommended.

Usually on the breaking day of the cleansing fast, the faster will find that the tongue after many days of producing mucus turns once again a fresh natural red color; the taste in the mouth turns sweet, bad breath and skin odor will have disappeared as all impurities and foul gases have finally left the body via the lungs and skin. He will find also that the urine becomes clear and has no odor, that the enema water passes out in a clean odorless foam and, most important of them all, is the return of natural hunger. This transition from fasting to hunger happens because the disease and waste matter and body supplies have been removed by autolysis, and at this point the body begins to consume its own healthy tissues and organs. The body's protective mechanism of instinct is reawakened and cries out for food. There is no fast too long and no damage can ever be done unless the faster is totally ignorant and purposely refuses to recognize the body's signals. Natural hunger will come to all persons who fast until their bodies become clean.

Not always do all of these signs appear together. But whether one or all appear, you can expect them all to soon follow each other. These are the signs that make one just sit down and say a prayer or do some meditation to give thanks to the higher energies for supplying the necessary strength that was needed for the purification of body and mind.

Not once has it been said that the entire process of a cleansing fast is simple; it does take perseverance to overcome food addiction. God was exact when He said, "we shall pay for our sins."

> *"And when all sins and uncleannesses are gone from your body, your breath shall become as pure as the breath of odorous flowers; your flesh as pure as the flesh of fruits reddening upon the leaves of trees; the light of your eye as clear and bright as the brightness of the sun shining upon the blue sky."* (Essene Gospel of Peace)

One intersting thing that occasionally happens during a fast is that people get so high from fasting that they do not want to come down. Many people at fasting clinics have to be talked into eating once again.

"Being forty days tempted of the devil. And in those days he did not eat nothing; and when they were ended, he afterward hungered." (St. Luke 4-2)

WILL I GAIN ALL MY WEIGHT BACK WHEN I START EATING AGAIN?

Once you begin to eat food again, you will naturally gain some weight back in water. Because of the sodium found in food, the body will retain fluid. This, however, is normal, but if you go back to or start eating too much of the wrong foods, you can expect the scale to rise.

The best method to keep your weight down is to just make fasting part of your life and begin to eat "lighter" foods. (See Chapter 13).

CHAPTER 11

HOW TO BREAK THE FAST

Whether you have been on a long fast or a short fast, do not break the fast with solid food as your first meal. It is very dangerous to break a fast with solid food as the food might rot in the intestinal tract. The body, in most cases, cannot digest it at this time of refeeding. Peristaltic action has to become accustomed to food again gradually. If the peristaltic action of the small intestines completely fails, the food will become impacted and can cause serious problems and even death.

On a Fast of Under Five Days

As you had to prepare to stop eating, now more importantly you must prepare to start eating. This is the most crucial time of the entire cleansing and healing process of the fast. Whether your fast turns out to be a success or failure depends on ending it correctly.

Even an idiot can fast but it takes intelligence and wisdom to break a fast right. Fasting from five to forty days, your stomach and intestines contract. As you get ready to break, you must do it slowly and only with juices. On a fast under five days, the faster can use his own judgement upon breaking, however, even he should for the first day drink only the juices of grapefruit, pineapple, tomato, grape, cantaloupe, watermelon, strawberry, and the juice of any other juicy fruits. These juices should be consumed at room temperature for easier digestion. On the second and third days eat lightly with vegetables or fruits. No meats, or heavy foods should be consumed.

On the Fast of Over Five Days

Take a day of juices for every five days of fasting. This is the rule to be followed whether the fast is five days or five months (there is a recorded fast in a case of obesity of 397 days). A fast of forty days requires eight days of juice consumption before solid food is safe. Do not drink fresh, alive juices during this time. Fresh juices are too active with enzymes for a stomach that has been deeply asleep for many days. Fresh juices will wake up the stomach villi too rapidly, shocking the system and causing much discomfort.

On the First Day of Breaking a Fast of Over Five Days
Cook Your Juices

If you use freshly squeezed juices, lightly cook or simmer them for ten to fifteen minutes then cool to body temperature. Heating stills the enzyme action of live food and in the stomach's arrested condition this is necessary to avoid shock.

Use Pure Juices

If possible, use only freshly squeezed orange or grape juice. Oranges are usually obtainable year around, but since grapes are only seasonal, you may buy any bottled pure grape juice and use it without cooking, pasteurization has already killed the enzymes, but make sure that the label says "unsweetened."

Dilute and Strain the Juices

After cooking; strain and dilute the juice with an equal part of distilled water, half and half.

Sip the Juice

After you have squeezed, cooked, strained and diluted

your juice, do not gulp down a whole glass or even half a glass. Introduce the juice slowly by taking two small sips every hour for the first three hours.

After sipping for three hours, increase the juice intake to two small swallows every hour for the next three hours. Next, proceed with one cup every hour until bedtime. Drink no more than one half a diluted gallon of juice on the breaking day. Remember, take in this fashion one day of juice for every five days that you have fasted. A fast of fourteen days requires three days of juices. On the third day you may begin to drink juice undiluted but still cooked.

BREAKING THE 21-40 DAY FAST

. . . Follow instructions for the first day of breaking the fast of over five days.

. . . The first two days drink cooked diluted juice before beginning the undiluted juices.

. . . On the third and fourth day of breaking a long fast you may begin to drink the juices whole but still cooked.

. . . Then on the fifth and sixth days you may begin to drink a vegetable broth or vegetable juice, but still cooked.

. . . The seventh and eighth days begin to drink raw uncooked vegetable or fruit juice but do not combine them. Drink vegetable juice two hours apart from fruit juice.

. . . During these eight days do not consume any heavy drinks, such as egg nog, milk shakes, kefir, smoothies, etc.

Chew Your Juices

In order to mix the valuable digestive juices and saliva necessary for the reawakening of the stomach, chew your juices just like solid food.

After you have properly awakened the stomach with juices, you may begin to introduce steamed fruits or vegetables. Do not eat any heavy protein, fried foods, or heavy starches. After the juice diet the first meal should be small and very easy to digest.

This food must be chewed slowly and thoroughly. The digestive process begins in the mouth. Stay on cooked fruits and vegetables for a period of three days before eating them raw. Gradually the body can return to a normal diet.

INTESTINAL FLORA

In the colon live a large amount of bacteria, most of which are harmless. These tiny little workers help move the contents of the colon along by digestion and fermenting, counteract adverse effects of putrefaction, (the cause of many diseases) and manufacture vitamins in the intestines.

Just as the roots of plants take their nourishment from the soil, so man's intestines take nourishment from his food. And just as many bacteria in the soil help nourish the plants, so man needs bacteria to provide him with proper nourishment.

These bacteria are called intestinal flora and are relatively harmless provided they stay in the intestines where they belong. However, if you should get these bacteria into your mouth — either by not properly cleaning your hands after going to the toilet or by drinking water contaminated with sewage, they can make you seriously ill.

The presence of a large amount of "good" bacteria will interfere with the growth of putrefactive bacteria and acts as a protection against invading organisms. Sometimes "bad" bacteria, (putrefactive bacteria) can crowd out the "good" bacteria. This overpowering occurs often because of a poor diet of meat, sugar, and chemicals, but when given a natural diet, the good bacteria will once again thrive and become dominant. Meat is the food that most often displaces the good bacteria.

The destruction of good bacteria can lead to serious symptoms of autointoxification and vitamin deficiencies. The good bacteria is also destroyed by the use of antibiotics, (e.g., penicillin). White sugar and sugar products even in small percentages can destroy the good bacteria also. Antibiotics may eradicate the cause of an infection but they certainly also destroy the vitamin producing good bacteria which then have to be replaced. A long fast also sterilizes the colon, especially when regular enemas and colonic irrigations are used.

After food is again introduced into the system it is very important to eat some fermented foods which contain the natural lactic acid producing bacteria.

Fermentation is the process by which bacteria is produced in foods. During the process of fermentation, the natural lactic acid is produced which is extremely important in providing a medium for beneficial bacterial growth. Fermented foods can be thought of as pre-digested foods.

Some of the most common foods eaten that are high in lactic acid producing bacteria are yogurt, sauerkraut, sour pickles, sour milk and fermented grains and green vegetables.

Without properly providing a medium for the growth of lactic acid producing bacteria after fasting, constipation resulting in putrefaction can occur corrupting the entire body. The colon will become full of putrefactive matter decreasing the benefits of the fast. A clean intestinal tract is the key to health. Do not give waste a chance to slow down or stop as it moves through the intestintes.

WHEN WILL I HAVE MY FIRST BOWEL MOVEMENT?

Do not worry if you do not immediately have a bowel evacuation. It often takes the system a day or two to adjust once again to eating and the disposing of waste.

Some people, however, will have an evacuation shortly after eating the first meal, but since elimination is different for each person, I cannot predict the time of your first movement. As you begin to eat foods that stimulate the peristaltic motion of the bowels, you will again establish a regular and natural system for elimination of waste products. The bowels, like the stomach, need regularity and will accustom themselves to work at a certain time of the day, provided you get on a good diet and get plenty of exercise. A rebuilding diet of natural, largely raw food should be employed to prevent future illness, obesity, and the cluttering of your system and as a continuing way of eating.

CHAPTER 12

AFTER THE FAST

In the preceeding chapters we dealt with the cleansing and purification of the body and now in these last chapters I will suggest a cleaner way of eating in the future which if sincerely followed will keep you slim, healthy and prevent you from having to repeat so intense a cleansing process.

Since this book is written as a complete guide for fasting and should be used as a reference throughout your fast, I will not present what alot of other fasting books do, that is a lot of tempting dishes and recipes. That would only make it harder for the faster as he thumbs through the pages. I will, though, talk about the bad foods, what should be eliminated, and what natural product can replace it. You will not only read what not to eat but be glad that you are fasting to clean out what you have eaten. As we learned in the second chapter death and disease frequently begin in the colon with the putrefaction and the rotting of unfit foods which produces the impure and undesireable bacterial matter that corrupts the entire organism. We must begin to recognize that a diet of uncooked natural fruits, vegetables, seeds, some nuts and grains is the key to a clean, healthy, balanced body.

Today's meals are incorrectly balanced. People consume too many chemicals and additives, they eat too much, too quickly, and too often. Their meals are overcooked, improper combinations causing obesity, digestive problems and other associated diseases. When someone asks me, "Well what is the ideal diet?" I usually reply with "Whatever is fresh, wholesome, and natural that goes into the body and comes out the quickest and easiest leaving an odorless stool." That is foods that have been proven by experience to digest and assimilate faster and more easily. Roughage in the form of fresh fruits, sprouts, and vegetables are good examples of these foods. For many it is very hard to eat only these foods as today's modern man has been raised essentially on junk and overcooked devitalized foods. It is very hard even for the strictest health nut to honestly say that he's sickened by the taste of, say pies and cakes. Most youngsters, before much conditioning to speak of has taken place, love the tastes of sweets and know no better than to eat them. They do taste good but even arsenic tastes good. That is why the bugs eat it. However, when a man enjoys his sense of taste, to the neglect of his intellect, he destroys his body. Man, the greatest thinking animal, is his own worst enemy and has proven many times over his ability to harm himself in spite of knowing better. Most Americans will not eat a diet of fresh raw vegetables, fruits and grains but at least they should cut down on cooked and junk foods gradually learning to replace them with at least seventy five percent raw fruits, sprouts and vegetables and to fast one or two days a week to clean out the other twenty five percent of junk they continue to consume.

VISIT A HEALTH FOOD STORE

All that I can do here is suggest what is healthy and what is not. It's up to you to adopt a good diet and investigate nutrition further. If you have not been to a health food store yet, it's time for the first visit. The clerks in most health food stores will be more than glad to serve and assist you. Shopping in health food stores is far more pleasant and personal than shopping in the super big stores which often are understaffed to where it is difficult to find a clerk, especially one who knows about food and nutrition. Also, you will be doing yourself a great disservice if you pass up all of the books on nutrition and health. There is usually a great deal of knowledge on the book shelves of health food stores. In nutrition a small amount of learning can be a dangerous thing, but it only takes a little time and a few good books to be well into the area of nutrition and very quickly able to direct yourself.

After fasting foods such as meat, coffee, soda pop, alcohol, corn twirls, potato chips, sugared breakfast cereals, etc. will not seem as delightful as before. Natural foods will seem more inviting as the body can digest and assimilate them more easily.

After starting out with a clean system and eating natural foods, you will eat smaller amounts of food than before, because the body gets better nourished with less food. More nutrients become available and are better assimilated when raw natural foods are eaten. It's not the food the body wants but nourishment. People are not nourished by the amount of food they eat but in proportion to how much they digest and assimilate. This is why thin people who have trouble gaining weight should fast. Thin people can gain weight faster and easier when the organs of digestion and assimilation are in good working condition. Eating fat, starch, and sweets to gain weight only defeats the purpose. So the secret to gaining weight lies in the rejuvenation of the digestive and assimilative system.

Through fasting you often correct many wrong eating patterns and have no desire to return to them. After fasting you will have learned and can accept the fact that it is not the amount of food that you eat, but rather the kind of food and its quality that is important.

After a fast you are faced with either putting junk back in a clean body or starting a whole new regime of eating cleaner foods. Which will it be? Are you going to continue eating toxic and fat meats, greasy fried foods, pastry products and bread made from sugar and white flour that go in and never seem to come out? Or are you willing to begin to consider changing your diet to the eating of as much raw food as you like, supplementing your diet with fresh raw vegetables and fruit juice?

Everything is always subject to change, so why not your diet? Another law of nature is that we all evolve at different speeds. The change to a better diet can be made immediately or gradually. But as long as you are going forward toward a cleaner diet and not backward toward sickness you are doing well. Good eating and health can become one of the best liked and most worthwhile hobbies you and your family or friends have ever had.

Make up your mind that you want it, and set your mind to get it. This is the first and most important step to better health. So many people say "Why the bother, I'm going to die sooner or later anyway." Sure you are going to die, but it's the idea of being stricken with disease or cancer and bedridden twenty years before and up to the time of your death. Who wants to die a slow miserable death? Man's body is meant happily to live to a ripe old age and then to pass on during sleep of peaceful causes. We also are on this earth to do spiritual work. I feel that the more time I have the more I will get done.

There is no drug, nor person who can make you eat better. You are the only person who can do that. Books and teachers can help but patience, persistence and will power are needed. Take the necessary time required, but remember a move forward is a move for the better. Along the way, if you desire some junk food or desire meat badly, eat it. It is better to go ahead and eat rather than toss it around in your head for hours wasting energy. But feel no guilt. Guilt will make you sicker than the food.

And do not accept any idea about health and nutrition without the scientific knowledge to back it up. Everything that I have written here is backed not only by authority but is also proved by the results of many cases.

WHY YOU SHOULD EAT MOSTLY LIVE FOODS

As food is cooked it is destroyed. Enzymes which are vital catalysts necessary for the proper digestion and assimilation of food are destroyed by heat. Heated food also destroys some of the gastric enzymes needed for digestion and can destroy up to seventy five percent of the available protein in most foods. In cooking, vitamins and minerals are also reduced and usually they get thrown out with the cooking water. If you don't believe cooking destroys the life in foods, cook a seed, then try to germinate it. It will not grow. Man is the only animal on this planet who destroys most of his food.

Raw fruits and vegetables act upon the digestive and alimentary canal as a cleansing agent thus eliminating and preventing constipation. Constipation causes obesity. Raw foods are easy to digest and pass through the normal system and are eliminated more quickly than cooked foods. Again, I say many people reared on cooked foods would find it difficult to eat only raw foods. But any effort taken toward the consumption of more raw foods is a step forward. At least seventy five percent of your diet should be alive and eaten in a raw state. If you do cook your food, avoid baking, broiling (upside down frying) and frying the foods. Instead lightly steam the food using little water. The trick to safe cooking is to not let the water touch the food while steaming.

There are, however, many vegetables such as potatoes, yams, celery, etc. that can tolerate some cooking without suffering too much damage.

> *"We are living in an age where eating lots of raw foods is essential. Cooking destroys many of the vitamins, all of the enzymes, chelated minerals, nucleic acids and chlorophyll. The heat disorganizes the protein structure, leading to deficiency of some of the essential amino acids. The lack of complete protein in the diet contributes to premature aging. If the diet is at least 80% raw this does not occur."* (Viktoras Kulvinskas)

THE MOVE TO A BETTER WAY OF EATING

Clean up your diet by starting to eliminate the bad meats, sugar and all foods made with sugar, and salt, (sodium Chloride), pasteurized dairy products, and all snack, canned, counter and processed or over-cooked foods, all white flour products, (breads, rolls, pastries), coffee, tea — unless Herbal — alcohol, chemical laden foods, and all unnecessary drugs and stimulants such as tranquilizers, aspirin, etc. All of this junk may satisfy a psychological craving but add little to our true physiological needs.

REPLACE	WITH
Refined White Sugar	Honey, date sugar, grape sugar, molasses (unsulphured) black strap molasses, maple syrup, clean raw sugar.
White Flour Products (White bread, pastries, etc.)	Whole wheat, rye, and barley (all bread should be eaten toasted to reduce the mucus that fresh bread forms)
Table Salt Sodium Chloride (contributing factor to many diseases and disorders, e.g. high blood pressure and fluid retention in the body)	Sea Salt (if used sparingly) Kelp or Dulse. (Salt is found naturally in most fruits and vegetables and other food-stuffs when they are eaten raw).
Dairy Products — Milk (heated or processed). Cheese, pasteurized Butter, Yogurt.	Non-pasteurized dairy products — Yogurt that is natural and plain without preserves and sweeteners — Raw milk or soya milk. rennetless cheese. All dairy products should be used sparingly.
Supermarket Breakfast Cereals.	Whole natural grain cereals that have been organically grown without sugar coating. They usually consist of barley, buckwheat, unbleached whole wheat, millet, rye and flax. Available in most food stores.
Coffee (too acid forming)	Can be replaced with an herbal coffee made from the root of the dandelion (no acid).
Tea (Caffeinated) (too acid forming)	Herbal Teas (no acid)
Soda Pop, Kool Aid and all imitation fruit drinks sweetened with sugar.	Freshly squeezed fruit juices or natural unsweetened bottled juices (juicers can be bought cheaply).
Red Meats (beef steak, etc.) Red meats contain h i g h amounts of uric acid.	If you must continue to eat meat, white meats, fish and foul are much cleaner meats.
Frozen and canned fruits and vegetables.	Fresh fruits and vegetables.

Fruits

Begin to replace all frozen and canned fruits with fresh or dried fruits. Soak dried fruits in water overnight before eating. Fresh fruit, the ideal food, should be used as a meal in itself as the acids in fruit do not combine well with other foods (see page 108). Fruits undergo little or no digestion in the mouth and stomach and are quickly sent to the intestines. Fruits are the plant's natural ovaries and contain its seeds. They were among the first foods of early man and contain vitamins A, B1, B2, C, niacin, choline, inositol, folic acid and are high in the bioflavanoids. Many minerals are also found in fruits, iron, copper, phosphorous, and sulphur as well as the easily assimilated simple sugars, fruit acids, and enzymes. Fruits are mostly eaten raw and are a better source of the water soluable vitamins than vegetables which are often cooked; and as we know cooking destroys these vitamins. The daily consumption of fruit is a digestive aid and they are low in calories.

Listed are the seasonal fruits available throughout the year in most stores thanks to modern shipping.

Apples
Apricots
(Fresh and dried (Unsulphured)
Avocados
Blackberries
Blueberries
Cantaloupes
Cherries (fresh, dried)
Cranberries
Currants
Dates
Figs (5 kinds fresh, dried unsulphured)
Grapefruit
Grapes
Honeydew Melons
(other melons)

Lemons and Limes
Mangos
Nectarines
Olives
Oranges
Papayas
Peaches (fresh, dried)
Pears (fresh, dried)
Pineapples (fresh, dried)
Pomegranates
Plums
Prunes (fresh, dried)
Raspberries
Strawberries
Tangerines
Tomatoes
Watermelon

Vegetables

Vegetables have been a part of the diet for most of us whether we are vegetarians or meat eaters. Vegetables include the green and leafy parts of plants (spinach, lettuces) the roots and tubers (carrots, radishes, potatoes, etc.) and the fruits (tomatoes, cucumbers, pumpkins) and the seeds (corn, etc.). Mushrooms are thought to be vegetables, but actually they are fungi.

Vegetables contain necessary vitamins and minerals. The fibers of raw vegetables (and fruits) promote intestinal motility and therefore are an aid to the absorption and utilization of nutrients. Again, cooking kills and reduces the effectiveness of food. Raw vegetables should be used in salads instead of cooking them. If at all possible, vegetables should be organic, and free from pesticides and sprays as all foods should be. Organically grown vegetables are available in some health food stores. A list of farmers who grow organically is usually available through the local farm bureau.

Listed are the different vegetables now also available most of the year.

Artichokes	Dandelion Greens
Asparagus	Dill
Beets (4 kinds)	Egg Plant
Brussel Sprouts	Endive
Cabbage	Escarole
Carrots	Garlic
Cauliflower	Green Peas
Celery	Kale
Chives	Leeks
Corn	Lettuce (6 kinds)
Cucumbers	Mustard Greens
Okra	Spinach
Onions	Squash
Parsley	String Beans
Parsnips	Swiss Chard

Potatoes (4 kinds)   Turnips
Green Peppers   Turnip Greens
Radishes   Watercress
Rhubarb   Yams

Nuts and Seeds

All nuts and seeds should be eaten raw and not roasted, toasted and salted. For easier chewing and digestion, nuts and seeds should be ground in a seed and nut grinding machine before eating, or chewed very well. Nuts and seeds are rich in protein and most nutritious when eaten from the shell.

Seeds are the ripened ovules of plants of the highest order. They contain the germ or embryo (the reproductive part of the seed) and the endosperm (containing the stored food material for the plant), and the outer cover or shell.

The size of seeds and nuts may range from as small as a dustlike particle to the size of the coconut, the largest seed. All seeds and nuts are highly nutritive and are rich in oil containing unsaturated fatty acids, Vitamin E and several vitamins of the B complex, minerals and proteins. Listed are the seeds and nuts.

NUTS

Acorns
Almonds
Cashew Nuts
Chestnuts
Coconut
Filberts or Hazel
Peanuts
Pecans
Pistachios

SEEDS

Alfalfa
Chia
Pumpkin
Sesame
Sunflower

Grains

The highly concentrated food grain is the seed of the grass. Its value for growth is apparent from its long use as the basic food in the raising of sturdy horses and cattle. With its proper use, strong and healthy people can be raised also.

Rye	Unpolished Rice
Oats	Corn
Whole Wheat	Pumpernickle
Barley	Millet

Legumes

The legumes (beans and peas) are another of man's first foods. They are all high in protein. When sprouted (or germinated) they increase their protein and change it into an even more readily digestible form as amino-acid.

	PEAS
Garbanzo	Dried peas
Kidney	Split peas
Lentil	Rye
Mung	Oats
Pinto	Whole Wheat
Soybeans	Barley

Herbs

Herbs, too, have been associated with man since his beginning. The name "herb" is commonly applied to all plants and their products, (roots, stems, leaves, flowers, seeds, and fruits), that are used for both medicinal quality or as seasoning in cooking. Any seed-producing annual, biannual, or perennial that has no woody stems and dies at the end of the season may be called an herbal plant.

Herbal teas are not only known to alleviate indigestion, constipation, etc., but also are quite tasty either hot or cold, sweetened or natural as a beverage.

"Remedies from chemicals and minerals will never stand in favorable comparison with the products of nature — the living cell of the plant, the final result of the rays of the sun, the mother of all life. When correctly used, herbs promote the elimination of waste matter and poisons from the system by simple, natural means. They support nature in its fight against disease; while chemicals, not being assimilable, add to the accumulation of morbid matter and only stimulate improvement by suppressing the symptoms." H.E. Kirschner, M.D.

Sprouting

Sprouts provide the cleanest, most nutritious and inexpensive food available.

- Sprouts can be grown in the middle of the city right in your own living room by anyone, even children.
- Sprouting is an excellent hobby for the entire family.
- Sprouts need no soil, sprays or insecticides and are free from bothersome bugs and insects.
- All that is needed are some seeds or grains, a mason jar, cheese cloth, and pure water.
- Sprouting takes only three days of growth before eating.
- Sprouts are inexpensive and can be used in snacks and in salads. A few ounces of alfalfa seed will produce enough sprouts for a family for two weeks at very little cost.

Sprouts are the immature outgrowth of the plant, or the shoot from its germinated seed. During the germination period, almost all of the nutritive values in the seeds increase.

Alfalfa, wheatberries, mung beans, radish, fenugreek, sunflower, chick pea, and many more can be sprouted and are available and organic from most health food stores. There are numberous books on the subject of sprouting, also available in health food stores.

104

Juicing

Fruit and vegetable juice can be easily extracted with the use of a juice extractor, better known as a juicer. All fresh juices are easily digestible and high in vitamins, minerals and enzymes. Fruit fuice gives instant energy because of the quickly digested fruit sugars. Commercial processed juices are usually fortified with vitamins and minerals and most often contain added sugar, preservatives and coloring agents. The nutritive value of all bottled and canned juices is reduced further because of the high temperature used to cook the juices while canning and pasteurizing. Raw juice is much healthier and recommended by nutritionists and doctors alike. There are many books in print on juice therapy as a correction for a lot of disorders and diseases.

Never Overeat

When food is eaten in large amounts much of it remains undigested and acts as a poison in the body causing the organism to become sluggish and heavy since you consume more food than your body needs or can use.

"Other equally serious mischiefs may arise from the accumulation in the system of a greater quantity of nutritive material than can be utilized, which occasions general clogging and obstruction of all the bodily functions, and imposes an enormous burden upon the kidneys in the elimination of unusable material."
(R.B. Pearson)

If people limited themselves to just the right amount of food, these conditions would never come about, and there would never be a need for fasting. Excess food will cause damage.

Furthermore, most compulsive eaters are always hungry

because they are undernourished. Remember, it is not the quantity but the quality of the food that is important. When nourishing food is consumed in small portions, the less hunger you will have because food is more efficiently digested, assimilated, and utilized.

Chew Your Food Well

Food should be chewed well and thoroughly insalivated because digestion begins in the mouth. The reason for proper chewing is both a mechanical (breaking down the food into small pieces) and a chemical process as well for saliva (ptyalin) is alkaline, and the first stage of digestion must happen in an alkaline medium (carbohydrates only).

If food is chewed and mixed properly with saliva, which comes from many small salivary glands located on the inside of the cheeks, the food itself is almost half digested before it enters the stomach. The stomach, remember, has no teeth. The enzymes in saliva start digesting certain foods while we chew and swallow them, and continue to do their work until destroyed by stomach acids. At this time the job is turned over to a stronger group of enzymes, pepsin in the presence of strong hydrochloric acid. The food then moves into the intestines (also alkaline) where nutrients are absorbed. In the small intestines other enzymes complete the preparation of the food material for assimilation into the body.

To eat in a hurry because of being late for work, or some other pressure is truly unwise, and it is far better to skip the meal completely than to swallow unchewed food.

Eat Only When Hungry

Try to discontinue eating by the clock — you most often fool yourself into eating just because the clock says breakfast, lunch, or dinner.

Begin to cut down on the size of breakfast and eventually discontinue it, thus extending the length of the nightly fast. Dr. Alvenia Fulton advises eating mini-meals, that is eating little meals only when hungry instead of big meals three or four times daily plus snacks.

"Never eat unto fullness" — Jesus

Proper Food combining

Often foods eaten together will interfere with the metabolism of each other. Proper food combining is just as important as eating good foods. There is ample evidence that every category of food requires a different enzyme for digestion. The ideal diet would be that of one food at a time, that is to eat only one food at any one meal. Most people will not do this; I don't, but I try to eat as few things together as possible and keep those few foods in the relatively same digestive categories.

Proper food combining will assure better nutrition as a result of better digestion, and it also gives protection against poisoning from improperly combined foods spoiling in the digestive tract. Foods that have rotted in the digestive track do not supply the body with vitamins.

Bad food combinations will not only distill poisons but cause bad breath from gastro-intestinal fermentation and putrefaction, gas in the abdomen, producing foul smelling stools, sleepless nights, constipation, the lack of appetite, nervousness, etc.

Following is a food combination chart compiled by the Hippocrates Health Institute. Learning to combine foods properly will result in a more balanced metabolsim.

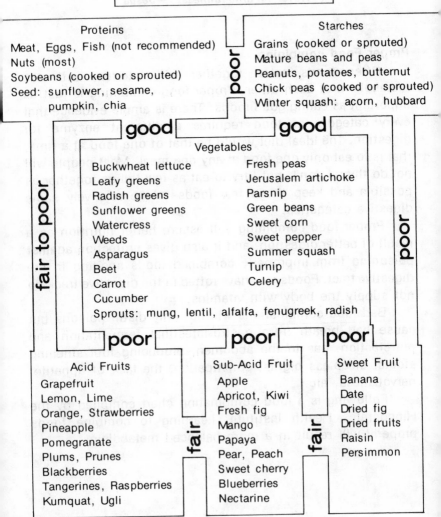

Food Combining For Easier Digestion

Proteins

Meat, Eggs, Fish (not recommended)
Nuts (most)
Soybeans (cooked or sprouted)
Seed: sunflower, sesame,
        pumpkin, chia

poor

Starches

Grains (cooked or sprouted)
Mature beans and peas
Peanuts, potatoes, butternut
Chick peas (cooked or sprouted)
Winter squash: acorn, hubbard

good   **good**

Vegetables

Buckwheat lettuce
Leafy greens
Radish greens
Sunflower greens
Watercress
Weeds
Asparagus
Beet
Carrot
Cucumber

Fresh peas
Jerusalem artichoke
Parsnip
Green beans
Sweet corn
Sweet pepper
Summer squash
Turnip
Celery

Sprouts: mung, lentil, alfalfa, fenugreek, radish

fair to poor   **poor**

poor   **poor**   **poor**

Acid Fruits

Grapefruit
Lemon, Lime
Orange, Strawberries
Pineapple
Pomegranate
Plums, Prunes
Blackberries
Tangerines, Raspberries
Kumquat, Ugli

Sub-Acid Fruit

Apple
Apricot, Kiwi
Fresh fig
Mango
Papaya
Pear, Peach
Sweet cherry
Blueberries
Nectarine

Sweet Fruit

Banana
Date
Dried fig
Dried fruits
Raisin
Persimmon

fair   **fair**

CHAPTER 13

CHANGING TO A LIGHTER DIET

Let me first explain what a vegetarian is. A person who calls himself a vegetarian will maintain a diet of fruits, vegetables, seeds, nuts grains and herbs. A person who adds to the diet of a vegetarian, milk, cheese, and eggs is call an "ovo-lacto vegetarian." A lacto vegetarian eats dairy products but excludes eggs. Then we have the person who eats only fruits who calls himself a "fruitarian." And of course, the meat eaters are called nothing or carnivorous. What I am concerned with here is vegetarianism. It is a much lighter diet that that of meats. Vegetarianism has proved its effectiveness not only in my life but also in many others. However, if you so desire, a lacto-vegetarian diet is not harmful providing you keep it down with eighty-five percent of your diet strictly vegetarian and the rest cheese, eggs or milk.

Vegetarianism is not new. It is as old as man. Both his physiological and spiritual history demonstrates his vegetarian nature. He has neither the teeth nor the short, straight digestive tract of the carnivore. Genesis states that the fruit trees are to be man's meat. Half of the world's population today is vegetarian. They eat no meat not only for health but also for spiritual reasons, like pacifism. The pacific refuse meat because they will not participate in the act of killing. It has been said that "Man just does not have the guts for eating meat."

Anthropologists point out that because of early man's inability to approach some animals without our modern weapons and his inability to catch others, he was forced to grow his own food or forage for it.

The teeth of meat eating animals are sharp fangs and they possess claws for the catching, tearing, and shredding of meat. Man has no fangs but rather possesses teeth only suitable for grinding and chewing.

> "It is my view that the vegetarian manner of living by its purely physical effect on the human body temperament would most beneficially influence the lot of mankind." (Albert Einstein, December 27, 1930)

In the Old Testament it is written in Genesis:

> "And the Lord planted a garden in Eden . . . And out of the ground made the Lord God to grow every tree that is pleasant to the sight, and good for food; And God said, Behold, I have given you every herb bearing seed which is upon the face of all the earth, and every tree . . . to you it shall be for meat."

The Hindus (noted for their closeness to God) attribute sanctity to cows. (The orthodox Jew prepared to die rather than eat the flesh of pigs.

The Pythagorean system of life required from its disciples abstinence from all flesh foods and recommended the use of such foods as fruit and nuts that need no cooking.

Even Moses through intuition, forbade the Jews to eat pork and did so to protect their health.

> "And the flesh of slain beasts in his body will become his own tomb. For I tell you truly, he who kills, kills himself, and whoso eats the flesh of slain beasts, eats of the body of death. For in his blood every drop of their blood turns to poison; in his breath their breath to stink; in his flesh their flesh to boils; in his bones their bones to chalk; in his bowels their bowels to decay; and their death will become his death."
> (Essene Gospel of Peace)

Cardinal Cooke of New York recently suggested that America should initiate one "meatless day" a week. If every American voluntarily fasted with no meat one day per week, this would be a fifteen percent reduction which would free fifteen million tons of grain that would have been used to feed cattle to feed the hungry. More than three times the food aid given by the U.S. for 1975 to underprivileged countries.

It takes not only the life from animals to feed foolish desires, but takes also fifty to one-hundred times more land to produce cows than it does to produce their equivalent in food as grains. Why not obtain your protein FIRST CLASS and eat the grain that builds the cows? Meat is a second rate protein.

> "Each pound of beef produced in American feedlots requires seven or eight pounds of grain that might otherwise be eaten by human beings rather than by animals." (Maya Pines, Breaking the Meat Habit)

J.M. Cowan points out a sad statistic in his book Nature, that "Since the Christian era one-hundred seven kinds of animals and almost one-hundred kinds of birds have been exterminated." However, in spite of all these facts, most Americans love the taste of the cow's ribs, or the T-Bone.

Since most people have been raised on heavy meats, it is hard to stop a life long habit. You cannot suddenly lose the appetite for meat unless you have deep, religious or philosophical reasons to help you along. Even if you become vegetarian for health reasons, it is hard to do it quickly. Every once in a while you will have the desire for meat when trying to quit. At this time it is better to go ahead and eat it and feel no guilt, for with a true and sincere desire for your own betterment, you will succeed. One of the world's leading nutritionist, Dr. Alvenia Fulton of Chicago, has stated that it takes 2 years of being a vegetarian before the desire for meat leaves entirely. Meat burns into an acid ash in the system and must be cleaned out. Through fasting and the use of herbs. you can quickly cleanse the system of uric acid and the toxemia which is caused by meat and gradually prepare to move into vegetarianism.

You will begin to notice better health even from the time you cut down on your meat intake. And it gets better as you eliminate meat entirely from the diet. Many people have been put in their grave in their prime (like the ribs) from heavy meat consumption, which is clearly linked to cancer, heart disease, and high blood pressure, just to name a few.

Animal flesh as well as fish and eggs all have the same thing in common, they decompose and putrefy rapidly inside the colon, generating virulent poisons and causing constipation and odorous stools.

The **Chicago Daily News,** Tuesday, January 15, 1975, in an article by the **Daily News Science** Editor, states that

"Fast rising cancer of the bowel is being blamed on too little roughage in the diet and too much beef. And that the high beef consuming countries, Denmark, Scotland, Argentina, Uruguay and the United States are also the countries with the fastest rising incidence of colon cancer."

"Not everybody who eats meat will develop cancer. It depends also on the body's inherent vitality, type of work, state of mind, choice of meat, amount of meat and other poisons in diet and environment." (Victoras Kulvinskas)

Most raw foods oxidize in the body into an alkaline ash while meats burn in the body, as I mentioned before, into an acid ash. The most healthy diet has been proven to be one on the alkaline side or "acid binding." Excess meat will cause problems in human livers where much of the meat is broken down before it can be used by the system.

The kidneys are overworked as they try to eliminate the excess poison from the rotting meat in the body and in the process they become injured. Uric acid is the by-product of meat that corrupts the tissues resulting in arthritis, rheumatism, gout and many more ailments including all types of nagging headaches. In short, every organ is harmed by the diet of meat, whereas on a diet of fruits, nuts, seeds and vegetables harm is not done.

Another simple reason not to eat meat is that you do not know how fresh the meat is that you are buying. Meat exposed even for a brief time quickly deteriorates.

The second the animal is slaughtered, his chemical laden flesh starts to decay. Because of chemicals, it is made to appear fresh. Without these added poisons, you would never want to eat it. You might want to start asking your butcher,

"How long has that piece been dead?" A fruit or vegetable in its natural state never lies, nothing is hidden, and doing without meat will also reduce the cost of weekly groceries by as much as fifty percent.

As you become a vegetarian, you must first learn how to get your proper protein.

You should learn just what vegetables and fruits should be eaten raw and what foods are more nutritious when cooked.

Sprouts are rated higher than beef in protein pound for pound. Tofu (soybean curd) is a Chinese dish of excellent protein. Dates are also excellent in protein. The Arabs used to cross the desert for days at a time getting their strength and protein only from dates and water. Six dates equals the protein of the best steak.

If vegetarianism did not supply the necessary proteins required for strength, then explain how Dick Gregory ran 2,980 miles on his Bicentennial Hunger Run of 1976 from Los Angeles to New York, New York across America at the age of forty four consuming no meat at all? In fact Mr. Gregory made that run without taking any solid food, averaging 50 miles each day!

In addition to learning about proteins, all the vitamins, minerals, enzymes, fats, sugars, and starches must become known. The new vegetarians must learn how to provide the proper balance of alkali and acid forming food. He also must learn proper food combining. Vegetarian diets are superior when care is taken in planning them. Vegetarianism should not be approached as a fad, but as a way of life. Become your own doctor. Study and learn and as in fasting, take it day by day, step by step. Remember, heavy meat consumption can be responsible for colonic disorders and "pot belly."

CHAPTER 14

HIGH PROTEIN DIET IS WRONG

The great fear that makes many Americans apprehensive about their daily diet is the threat about not getting enough protein. Those who are considering vegetarianism as a way of life face this issue.

Millions of dollars are being spent yearly on propaganda and advertisement by the livestock, dairy, and meat-packing industries promoting the belief that you need a high protein diet daily. It is no secret that these people are the ones who sponsor most of the research being done on your protein needs.

The more you buy meat and dairy products, the more these industries prosper. And you can well believe that their deceit will continue as long as we continue to buy their products. Most of America has been brainwashed by the meat and dairy lobby for over fifty years. We must begin to prevent the unnecessary suffering and constipation caused each year by diets of too much meat and dairy protein.

America eats more protein, especially meat, than any

other nation in the world today. Americans also have more heart disease, arthritis, cancer, obesity, high blood pressure, early death rate and miscarriages than any other country. Most of America's and Europe's recognized authorities and doctors in the field of nutrition and health promote low protein diets. The other doctors, those who urge high protein diets, know no better. They were taught little nutrition in medical school and they themselves are often examples of poor health. Medical training has already drifted dangerously far from the field of nutrition. There have been sufficient amounts of research done to destroy the high protein diet myth. Work by Dr. D.M. Hegsted of Harvard University, found that twenty-seven grams of protein is sufficient as compared to some of the figures that reach as high as one-hundred twenty grams a day. Dr. Hegsted's findings are proven around the world by many others all with findings that twenty-seven to fifty grams of protein daily is more than enough, with fifty grams completely sufficient for athletes and heavy workers. Most people also think that only meat will supply ample protein. This is also untrue. Protein consists of twenty-two amino acids of which nine are considered essential and cannot be produced within our bodies. These are: histidine (may be essential for children but not for adults), isoleucine, leucine, lysine, methionine, phenylalanine, threonine, tryptophan, and valine.

Our bodies are eighteen percent protein and every cell of it has to be built and rebuilt out of the twenty-two different kinds of acids. These amino acids come only from the food we eat however, not all foods contain all of the entire group of amino acids. The foods which lack one of more of the essential amino acids are called incomplete protein foods. Foods which contain all the essential amino acids are called complete protein foods. Based upon outdated research and enforced by the food industries, it was taken for granted that only animal proteins, fish, meat, eggs and dairy, contained complete proteins and that all vegetable proteins were incomplete. However, recent research backed by leading institutions, reveals that many fruits, vegetables, seeds, nuts and grains are excellent sources of complete proteins. Not only are these foods complete proteins but is has been established that vegetable proteins are higher in biological value than animal proteins and that raw, live proteins are superior to any cooked proteins. Your body can do better with less live proteins that it can with more cooked proteins.

Every vegetable, fruit, seed, nut and plant contains some protein, whether complete or incomplete. When the daily diet consists of these natural proteins, you do not have to worry about getting enough, for if one protein is incomplete, the other will usually balance it out. For example, one can mix rice (which is low in lysine), with beans (which are high in lysine) to make a high quality combination that far surpasses the protein value of either food alone. You also do not have to worry about the need to eat a complete protein mixture at any one meal. What is more necessary is your amino-acid intake for the day, week, or month.

It is very easy on a lacto-vegetarian diet to get too much protein, and on a meat diet when a person commonly eats everyting it is almost impossible not to get too much protein.

It is also a myth that you need to eat protein daily. You do need protein daily for the body but this does not mean that you have to eat it daily. Fasting has demonstrated that your body not only exists for weeks without food, but actually improves its condition when all food is excluded.

It is scientific knowledge that the albumin reading, (the level of protein in the blood) remains normal and steady during a short fast although no protein is taken at the time. Amino acids from old cells are reused for the building of new cells during fasting. People who strive to take heavy meat protein into their systems to get their "quota" should know that no proteins eaten in larger amounts that the acutal body needs, are stored in the body. They are oxidized, burned as fuel for energy. And as the process of burning excess flesh protein occurs, pathological residues of metabolic waste products are produced such as uric acid, urea, and others, all leading to toxemia.

Heavy meat eaters are prone to become "saturated" in different ways from this waste. This in turn decreases physical capabilities rather than increasing them as we have been led to believe. It is not at all uncommon for the athlete to eat a large beef steak to obtain energy before the contest and suddenly in the middle of the match drop out from exhaustion from its digestion and pains resulting from excess acid.

Too much protein in the diet also results in bacterial putrefaction of the intestines and destroys the necessary benign bacteria. This pollution is the prime cause of dark, toxic, foul smelling stools and foul breath. The increase protein intake, even from vegetable sources will result in an inverse ratio of germ efficiency. In the case of meat protein, an even more serious bacterial exchange can be expected. The production of good bacteria is not enough to overpower the increased proportions of toxins left over during the conversion of animal protein.

A high protein diet of any kind is as wrong as the misguided people who enforce it. The excessive amounts of protein, which are highly nitrogenous, plus a large amount of carbohydrate consumption create a highly oppressive burden on the heart and digestive organs. A low protein diet is far superior, more natural, and much easier on all of the organs of the body. Breast milk is much lower in protein than cow's milk and as the human infant matures, even the already small amount of protein in the mother's milk is reduced. Throughout the child's development the milk changes and by the sixth to eighth month the percentage of protein may decrease by as much as forty-five percent.

Most Americans are convinced that a high protein diet will give an abundance of strength. This is also untrue. The International Vegetarian Society States:

"Since our muscular tissues consist chiefly of protein, the early students of physiology believed that this constituent was the source of muscular energy. Today we know that during muscular work under rational nutrition there is only a slight increase in the excretion of nitrogen, yet a noticeable increase in the excretion of carbonic acid and in the absorption of oxygen. Muscular energy therefore is mainly derived from non-nitrogenous substances like sugar and starch as exists in natural foods. The oxidation of the elements of food usually takes place in the active tissues, but according to our present knowledge of matter, it does not seem to occur at the expense of protein in living cells."

So in essence a high protein diet **does not** give that strength which many say but instead puts a tax on the whole system as the body has to excrete all excess nitrogen, burdening the liver and kidneys which in turn puts a strain on the heart. Only the carbon contained in natural foods is used for energy. This is often seen as some athletes turn to honey for energy and mountain climbers carry chocolate bars and other non-nitrogenous foods for instant energy.

Some people know all this while others haven't even heard of it. Now you have and are faced with a new concept, the true concept in eating. Try it, and prove it to yourself. On a low protein diet you will feel lighter and have more energy. You will save money and enjoy a longer healthier life. Doing without meat will reduce the cost of your protein by as much as fifty percent. In fact, to get down to the normal protein level, most Americans have to start putting an effort out "not" to get too much rather than to get enough.

The need for a cleansing fast is directly related to the toxicity of one's body. Eat light, stay healthy.

Abramowski, O.L.M*, **Fruitarian Diet and Physical Rejuvenation.** (Natal, South Africa: Essence of Health Publishing Company).

Adolph, E.F., **Physiology of Man in the Desert.** (New York: Interscience Publishing, Inc., 1947).

Airola, P.O., **Are You Confused?** (Phoenix, Arizona: Health Plus, 1971).

How to Keep Slim, Healthy and Young with Juice Fasting. (Arizona: Health Plus, Publishing, 1971).

Allen, F.N., "Control of Experimental Diabetes by Fasting and Total Dietary Restriction," **Journal of Experimental Medicine,** 1920.

Bach, E., **Heal Thyself.** (Essex, England: the C.W. Daniel Company, Limited, 1931).

Bailey, A.A., **The Consciousness of the Atom.** (New York: Lucis Publishing Company, 1922).

Bassler, A., **Diseases of the Digestive system.** (Philadelphia: F.A. Davis Company, Publisher, 1922).

"The Fasting Cure Answered." **Month Cycle and Medical Bulletin,** 4.

Benedict, F.G., **A Study of Prolonged Fasting Publications.** (Washington: Carnegie Institution, 1915).

Bragg, Paul, **The Miracle of Fasting.** (California: Health Science, Publishing).

Buchinger, O.H.F., **About Fasting.** (91 St. Martin's Lane, London: Thorsons Publishing, Ltd., 1961).

Cannon, W.B., **Bodily Changes in Pain, Hunger, Fear, and Rage.** (Harper and Row, 1963).

The Mechanical Factors of Digestion. (New York: Longmans, Green and Company, 1911).

The Wisdom of the Body. (New York: W.W. Norton and Company, Inc., 1932).

Carlson, A.J., **The Control of Hunger in Health and Disease.** (Chicago: 1916).

Carrington, H., **Vitality, Fasting, and Nutrition.** (New York: Rebman Company, 1908).

Fasting for Health. (Mokelumne Hill, California: Health Research, 1953).

Cheifetz, P.M., "Uric Acid Excretion and Ketosis in Fasting, 14, 1965.

Cott, A., **Fasting—The Ultimate Diet.** (Bantam Books, Inc., 1975).

Cubberley, P.T., "Lactic Acidosis and Death After the Treatment of Obesity by Fasting." **New England Journal of Medicine, 272,** 1965.

Davenport, H.W., **Physiology of the Digestive Tract.** (Chicago: Year Book Medical Publishers, Inc., 1962).

De Vries, A., **Therapeutic Fasting.** (Chandler Book Company, 1963).

Dewey, E.H., **The No-Breakfast Plan and the Fasting Cure.** (London: L.N. Fowler and Company, 1900).

Du Bois, E.F., **Basal Metabolism in Health and Disease.** (Lea and Tibiger, 1936).

Editorial, "President Status of Heat Processing Damage to Protein Foods." **Nutrition Review, 8** (7) 193, 1950.

Ehret, A., **The Muscusless Diet Healing System.** (Beaumont, California: Ehret Literatire and Publishing Company, 1972).

Rational Fasting. (Beaumont, California: Ehret Literature and Publishing Company, 1975).

Enselme, J., **Unsaturated Fatty Acids in Atherosclerosis.** (Pergamon Press, 1962).

Ewald, E., **Recipes for a Small Planet.** Ballantine Books, 1973.

Frazier, B.C., "Prolonged Starvation," (Louisville), **Journal of Medicine and Surgery,** 15: 147-254, 1908.

Fryer, Lee, and Simmons, D., **A Dictionary of Food Supplements.** (New York: Mason/Charter, 1975).

Whole Foods for You. (New York: Mason and Lipscomb Publishing, 1974).

Fulton, A.M., **The Fasting Primer.** (C.A.M.S. Press).

Galdston, Iago, **Beyond the Germ Theory.** (New York, Minneapolis: Health Education Council Publishers, 1954).

Gamble, J.L., "Physiological Information Gained from Studies on the Life Raft Ration." **Harvey Lectures, 42,** 1946-47.

Garten, M.O., **The Health Secrets of a Naturopathic Doctor.** (West Nyack, N.Y.: Parker Publishing Company, Inc., 1967).

Gerson, M., **Cancer Therapy.** (N.Y.C.: Dura Books, Inc., 1958).

Gordon, "A Prolonged Fast." **Montreal Medical Journal,** 36-482, 1907.

Gregory D., **Dick Gregory's Natural Diet for Folks Who Eat; Cookin with Mother Nature.** (New York: Harper and Row).

Guelpa, A., **The Science of Human Life.** (New York: Fowler and Wells, 1843).

Guyton, A., **Physiology of the Body.** (Philadelphia: W.B. Saunders Company, 1964).

Gunn, R.A., **Forty Days Without Food.** (New York: Albert Metz and Company, 1880).

Hay, W.H., **Health via Food.** (East Aurora, New York: Sun-Diet Health Foundation, 1929).

Hazzard, L.B., **Fasting for the Cure of Disease.** (Physical Culture Publishing Company, 1910).

Howe, P.E., and Hawk, P.B., "A Metabolism Study on a Fasting Man." Proc. Am. Soc. Biol. Chem., 31, 1912.

Hunters, B.T., **Food Additives and Your health.** (New Canaan, Connecticut: Keats Publishing, Inc., 1972).

Jyotirmayananda, Swami, **The Way to Health and Happiness Through Hatha Yoga.** (San Juan, Puerto Rico, U.S.A., 1964).

Kallet, A., and Schlink, F.J., **100,000,000 Guinea Pigs.** (New

York: The Vanguard Press, Inc., 1933).

Kauz Herman, **Tai Chi Handbook.** (Garden City, New York: Doubleday and Company, Inc., 1974).

Keys, A., **The Biology of Human Starvation.** (University of Minnesota Press, 1950).

Kirschenbaur, H.G., **Fats and Oils.** (New York: Reinhold Publishing Corporation, 1944).

Kirschner, H.E., **Nature's Healing Grasses.** (California: H.C. White Publications, 1960).

Kloss, J., **Back to Eden.** (Santa Barbara, California: Lifeline Books, 1972).

Kulvinskas, V., **Love Your Body.** (Wethersfield, Connecticut: O'Mangod Press, 1972).

Survival Into the Twenty-First Century. (Wethersfield, Connecticut: O'Mangod Press, 1975).

Langefield, H.S., **Psychophysiology of a Prolonged Fast.** Psychological Monograph, 16:5, 1914.

Lapp'e, F.M., **Diet for a Small Planet,** (Ballentine Books, 1975).

Lerza, C., and Jacobson, M., **Food for People Not for Profit.** (New York: Ballantine Books, 1975).

Locke, D.M., **Enzymes—The Agents of Life.** (New York: Crown Publishers, Inc.).

Loewi, Otto, **From the Workshop of Discoveries.** (University of Kansas Press, 1953).

Long, C.N., "Studies on Experimental Obesity." **Journal of Endocrinology** (British) 15, VI, 1957.

Madfadden, B.A., **Fasting for Health,** (Madfadden Publications, 1923).

Macia, R., **The Natural Foods and Nutrition Handbook.** (New York: Harper and Row Publishing, 1972).

Man-Ch ing, Cheng, and Smith, W.R., **Tai-Chi.** (Vermont: Charles E. Tuttle Co., 1967).

Manocha, S.L., **Malnutrition and Retarded Human Development.** (Springfield, Illinois: Charles C. Thomas Publishing, 1972).

McCay, C.M., "Prolonging the Life Span." **Sci. Monthly, Vol. 139, 1934.**

McConkey, B., "The Effects of Wasting of Body Water." **Clin. Sci., 18, 1959.**

McEachen, J., **Fasting for Better Health.** (Escondido, Calif.: J. McEachen, 1957).

Meyers, A.W., "Some Morphological Effects of Prolonged Inanition." **Journal of Medical Research, '36: 51-77. 1917.**

Mills, C.A., **This Air We Breathe.** (Boston: The Christopher Publishing House, 1962).

Morgulis, S., **Fasting and Undernutrition.** (E.P. Dutton and Company, 1924).

Newman, L., **Make Your Juicer Your Drug Store.** (P.O. Box 368, Beaumont, California: Beneficial Books).

Null, B., **Biofeedback, Fasting and Meditation.** (New York: Pyramid Books, 1974).

Oldfield, J., **Fasting for Health and Life.** (London: C.W. Daniel Company, 1924).

Pearson, R.B., **Fasting and Man's Correct Diet.** (Mokelumne Hill, California: Health Research, 1921).

Penny, F., "Notes on a Thirty-Day's Fast." **British Medical Journal, 1, 1414-16, 1909.**

Prevention, "Eat Less to Live More." October, 1973.

Purinton, E.E., **The Philosophy of Fasting.** (New York: Lust Publishing, 1906).

Pyke, M., **Food and Society.** (London: John Murry, Publishing, 1968).

Shelton, H.M., **Fasting for Renewal of Life.** (Chicago, Illinois: Natural Hygiene Press, 1974).

Food Combining Made Easy. (San Antonio, Texas: Dr. Shelton's Health School, 1951).

The Hgyienic System, Vol. 3. (San Antonio, Texas: Dr. Shelton's Health School, 1934).

Sinclair, U.P., **The Fasting Cure.** (M. Kennerly, 1913).

Spencer, H., "Changes in Metabolism in Obese Persons During Starvation." **American Journal of Medicine, 40, 1966.**

Spencer, R.P., **The Intestinal Tract.** (Springfiled, Illinois: Charles Thomas Publishing, 1960).

Sweet, M.P., **Hints on Fasting Well.** (Mokelumne Hill, Calif.: Health Research, 1956).

Szekely, E.B., **The Essene Gospel of Peace.** (3085 Reynard Way, San Diego, California: Academy Books, Publishing, 1974).

The Therapeutics of Fasting. (Tecate, 1942).

Tannahill, R., **Food in History.** (New York: Stein and Day Publishing, 1973).

The International Vegetarian Society, **Man Heal Thyself.** (Chicago, Illinois: The International Vegetarian Society, 1975).

Troy, M.T., **Better Bowel Health.** (New York: Pyramid Books, 1974).

Walker, N.W., **Raw Vegetable Juices.** (New York: Pyramid Communications, Inc. 1972).

Welsh, A.L., **Side Effects of Anti-Obesity Drugs.** (Springfield, Illinois: Charles Thomas Publishing, 1962).

Williams, R.J., **Nutrition Against Disease.** (New York, Toronto, London: Pitman Publishing Corporation, 1971).

Winslow, A., and Herrington, L.P., **Temperature and Human Life.** (Princeton, New Jersey: Princeton University Press, 1949).

Winter, R., **Poison in Your Food.** (New York: Crown Publishers, Inc.)

Yogendra, Shri, **Yoga Personal Hygiene.** (Denver, Colorado: Nutri-Books).

Young, V., and Scrimshaw, N., "The Physiology of Starvation." **Scientific American,** October, 1971.

Zubiran, S., "Endocrine Disturbances and Their Dietetic Background in Undernourished Mexico." **Ann. Int. Med., 4,** 1954.

Index

Index

Index

TIPS FOR A SUCCESSFUL FAST

- Imagine hungry folks in places where the villages are entirely owned by landlords who decide what will be grown. Where the hungry work all day in the fields and still are unable to earn enough to feed themselves, let alone their families.

- Imagine a life without refrigerators, markets, bread boxes or cookie jars — Where each meal time is spent praying instead of eating.

- Imagine folks having to tell their babies or their mothers, "There is no food today."

- So imagine you are they. Close your eyes for just one minute and try to feel their pain and hear their cries. Find out just how attached you are to your constant availability of food. Then open your eyes and say to yourself out loud: **"I CAN FAST"** and **"I WILL FAST."**

To order additional copies of
THE LAYMAN'S GUIDE TO FASTING AND LOSING WEIGHT*
send us your name, address and $3.95 plus 75¢ (to help defray
postage and handling costs) to:

Sprout Publications, Dept. E,
5241 Ocean Blvd., Sarasota, Fl. 33581

Mr. / Mrs. / Miss _____

(please print)

Address _____

City _____ State _____ Zip _____

If you know someone who would benefit by fasting, send
them a copy of **THE LAYMAN'S GUIDE TO FASTING and
LOSING WEIGHT,** or just give us their names and addresses
and we'll contact them.

Mr. / Mrs. / Miss _____

(please print)

Address _____

City _____ State _____ Zip _____

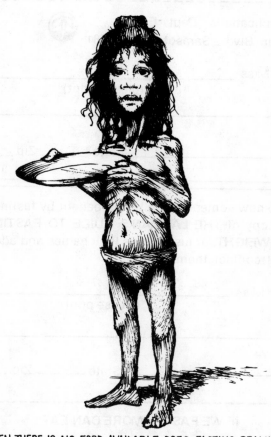

"ONLY WHEN THERE IS NO FOOD AVAILABLE DOES FASTING REALLY HURT."

131

To order additional copies of

THE LAYMAN'S GUIDE TO FASTING AND LOSING WEIGHT*

send us your name, address and $3.95 plus 75¢ (to help defray postage and handling costs) to:

Sprout Publications, Dept. E,
5241 Ocean Blvd., Sarasota, Fl. 33581

Mr. / Mrs. / Miss _____
(please print)

Address _____

City _____ State _____ Zip _____

If you know someone who would benefit by fasting, send them a copy of **THE LAYMAN'S GUIDE TO FASTING and LOSING WEIGHT,** or just give us their names and addresses and we'll contact them.

Mr. / Mrs. / Miss _____
(please print)

Address _____

City _____ State _____ Zip _____

IF WE FAST — MORE CAN EAT